Sleep Well

Editor: Danielle Lobban

Volume 465

AF854148

independence
educational publishers

First published by
Independence Educational Publishers
The Studio, High Green
Great Shelford
Cambridge CB22 5EG
England

www.independence.co.uk

© Independence 2025

Copyright

This book is sold subject to the condition that it shall not, by way of trade or otherwise, be lent, resold, hired out or otherwise circulated in any form of binding or cover other than that in which it is published without the publisher's prior consent.

Photocopy licence

The material in this book is protected by copyright. However, the purchaser is free to make multiple copies of particular articles for instructional purposes for immediate use within the purchasing institution. Making copies of the entire book is not permitted.

ISBN-13: 978 1 86168 925 2

Printed in Great Britain

Printed and bound by the Pureprint Group using its environmental print technology, a low-carbon, low-waste independently audited process that reduces environmental impact using 100% renewable energy, vegetable-oil-based inks and no industrial alcohol. 98% of all dry waste and 95% of press cleaning solvents are recycled. Pureprint are ISO 14001, EMAS and FSC certified and holds the Queen's Award for Enterprise: Sustainable Development.

EU Authorised Representative: Easy Access System Europe – Mustamäe tee 50, 10621 Tallinn, Estonia
Web: www.easproject.com Email: gpsr.requests@easproject.com

MIX
Paper | Supporting responsible forestry
FSC® C022913

Acknowledgements

The publisher is grateful for permission to reproduce the material in this book. While every care has been taken to trace and acknowledge copyright, the publisher tenders its apology for any accidental infringement or where copyright has proved untraceable. The publisher would be pleased to come to a suitable arrangement in any such case with the rightful owner.

The material reproduced in **issues** books is provided as an educational resource only. The views, opinions and information contained within reprinted material in **issues** books do not necessarily represent those of Independence Educational Publishers and its employees.

Although every effort has been made to ensure that website addresses are correct at time of going to press, Independence Educational Publishers cannot be held responsible for the content of any website mentioned in this book.

Images

Cover image courtesy of iStock. All other images courtesy of Freepik, Pixabay, Pexels, and Unsplash.

Additional acknowledgements

With thanks to the Independence team: Janey Hills, Klaudia Sommer and Jackie Staines.

Danielle Lobban

Cambridge, September 2025

Contents

Introduction

Sleep Well is volume 465 in the **issues** series. The aim of the series is to offer current, diverse information about important issues in our world, from a UK perspective.

About *Sleep Well*

Did you know humans spend a third of their life asleep? *Sleep Well* explores why sleep matters, how it affects your brain and mood, and what you can do to sleep better. Discover simple tips to take charge of your sleep and boost your wellbeing.

Our sources

Titles in the **issues** series are designed to function as educational resource books, providing a balanced overview of a specific subject.

The information in our books is comprised of facts, articles and opinions from many different sources, including:

- Newspaper reports and opinion pieces
- Website factsheets
- Magazine and journal articles
- Statistics and surveys
- Government reports
- Literature from special interest groups.

A note on critical evaluation

Because the information reprinted here is from a number of different sources, readers should bear in mind the origin of the text and whether the source is likely to have a particular bias when presenting information (or when conducting their research). It is hoped that, as you read about the many aspects of the issues explored in this book, you will critically evaluate the information presented.

It is important that you decide whether you are being presented with facts or opinions. Does the writer give a biased or unbiased report? If an opinion is being expressed, do you agree with the writer? Is there potential bias to the 'facts' or statistics behind an article?

Activities

Throughout this book, you will find a selection of assignments and activities designed to help you engage with the articles you have been reading and to explore your own opinions. Some tasks will take longer than others and there is a mixture of design, writing and research-based activities that you can complete alone or in a group.

Further research

At the end of each article we have listed its source and a website that you can visit if you would like to conduct your own research. Please remember to critically evaluate any sources that you consult and consider whether the information you are viewing is accurate and unbiased.

Issues Online

The **issues** series of books is complemented by our online resource, Issues Online.

On the Issues Online website you will find a wealth of information, covering over 75 topics, to support the PSHE and RSE curriculum.

Why Issues Online?

Researching a topic? Issues Online is the best place to start for...

Librarians

Issues Online is an essential tool for librarians: feel confident you are signposting safe, reliable, user-friendly online resources to students and teaching staff alike. We provide multi-user concurrent access, so no waiting around for another student to finish with a resource. Issues Online also provides FREE downloadable posters for your shelf/wall/table displays.

Teachers

Issues Online is an ideal resource for lesson planning, inspiring lively debate in class and setting lessons and homework tasks.

Our accessible, engaging content helps deepen students' knowledge, promotes critical thinking, and develops independent learning skills.

Issues Online saves precious preparation time. We wade through the wealth of material on the internet to filter the best quality, most relevant and up-to-date information you need to start exploring a topic.

Our carefully selected, balanced content presents an overview and insight into each topic from a variety of sources and viewpoints.

Students

Issues Online is designed to support your studies in a broad range of topics, particularly social issues relevant to young people today.

There are thousands of articles, statistics and infographs instantly available to help you with homework, research, and assignments.

With 24/7 access using the powerful Algolia search system, you can find relevant information quickly, easily and safely anytime from your laptop, tablet or smartphone, in class or at home.

Visit issuesonline.co.uk to find out more!

issues online
resources for schools, colleges & libraries

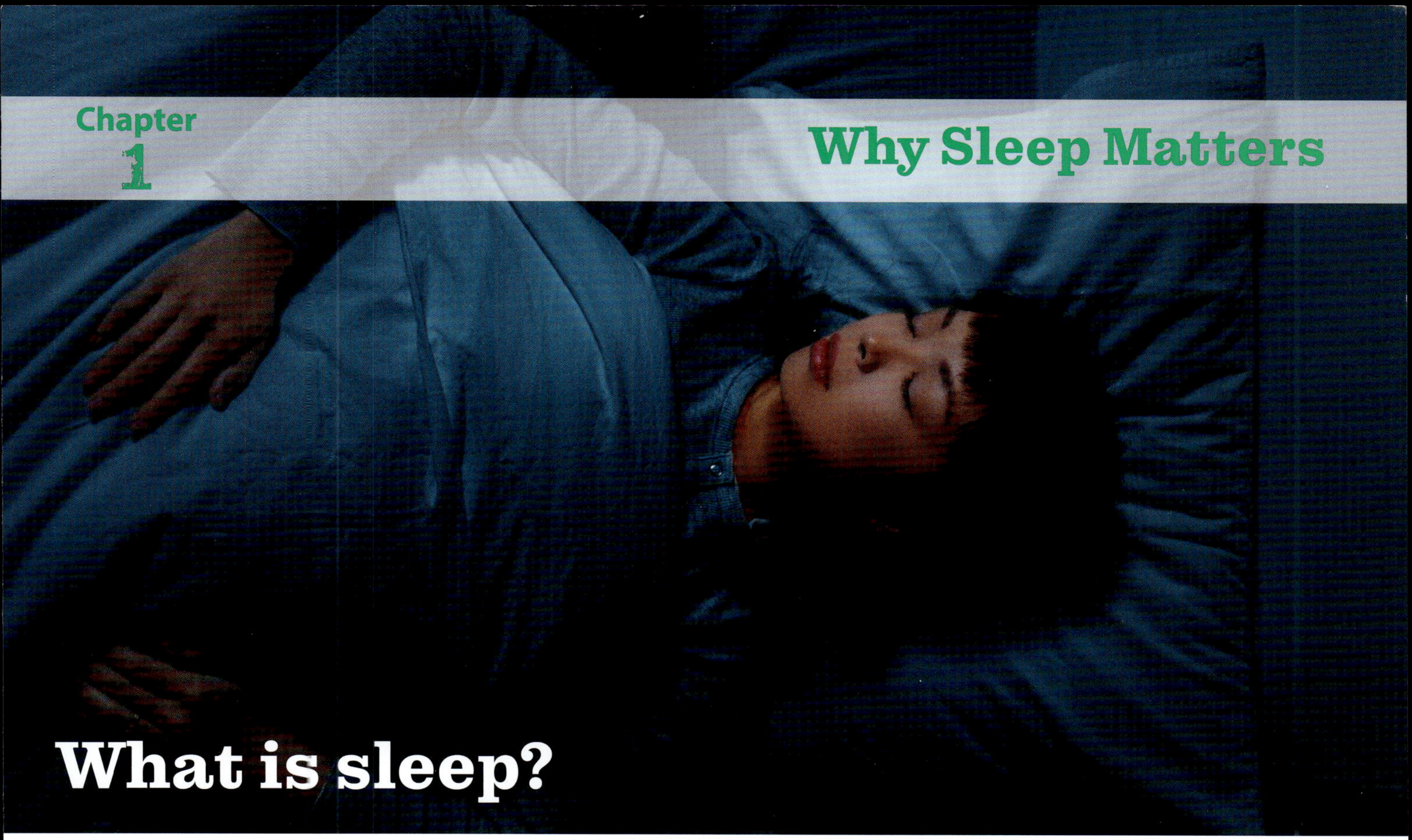

What is sleep?

Sleep is a universal human experience, yet it remains one of life's greatest mysteries. On average, we spend around twenty-six years asleep – roughly one third of a typical lifespan – and paradoxically another seven years simply trying to fall asleep. Despite this substantial investment of time, many of us underestimate just how vital sleep is for our physical health, mental wellbeing and overall quality of life.

Why sleep matters

From the moment we close our eyes to the instant we awaken, a complex series of biological processes unfolds. Sleep is not inactivity; it is a dynamic state during which body and mind undergo essential restorative work. Physically, sleep supports tissue repair, muscle growth and immune function. Mentally, it consolidates learning, strengthens memories and helps regulate emotions.

Every day, drowsiness impairs judgement, slows reaction times and undermines decision-making. Indeed, tired drivers are significantly more likely to make errors and cause road traffic collisions. Chronic sleep deprivation has even been weaponised as a form of torture – a stark reminder that lack of sleep can inflict profound damage on the human psyche.

Consequences of sleep deprivation

Short-term effects

The impact of inadequate sleep goes well beyond mere daytime drowsiness. In the immediate aftermath of a restless night, you may experience lapses in concentration, heightened irritability and impaired judgement that can lead to risk-taking behaviours. Even a single night of poor rest can affect reaction times and decision-making, increasing the likelihood of accidents and mistakes.

Long-term health risks

When sleep debt accumulates over weeks or months, its consequences become more serious. The immune system grows less effective, leaving you more vulnerable to infections and prolonging recovery periods. Chronic sleep loss is also associated with sustained elevations in blood pressure and a greater incidence of migraines and seizure disorders.

Mental health implications

Persistent sleep deprivation can profoundly affect psychological wellbeing. People who chronically miss out on sleep face a higher risk of developing depression and often experience exacerbated symptoms of anxiety. Cognitive functions such as memory retention and emotional regulation suffer, contributing to a vicious cycle of stress and insomnia.

Cardiometabolic consequences

Research has linked enduring sleep restriction to an increased likelihood of cardiovascular disease and metabolic disorders, including type 2 diabetes and obesity. Disruptions to hormonal balance – particularly those governing appetite and glucose metabolism – mean that skimping on sleep can also lead to weight gain and insulin resistance over time.

Use as a form of torture

Sleep deprivation has been employed as a coercive technique, whereby individuals are forcibly kept awake for extended periods – sometimes days at a time – to prevent rest or dreaming. Deprived of sleep, the mind and body begin to deteriorate: confusion sets in, hallucinations may occur, mood swings intensify and the boundary between reality and illusion can blur. This method is designed to wear a person down until they comply with demands. International law deems sleep deprivation for coercion illegal and classifies it as cruel, inhuman and degrading treatment.

Key functions supported by sleep

Sleep facilitates a host of vital physical and psychological processes:

Learning and memory – the brain consolidates new information during sleep, transforming fragile short-term memories into stable, long-term ones.

Emotional regulation – sufficient sleep helps us process emotions, reducing irritability and building resilience.

Decision-making and problem-solving – a well-rested mind assesses risks more accurately and arrives at sound conclusions.

Energy conservation – sleep lowers metabolic demand, preserving fuel for wakeful hours.

Growth and healing – deep sleep triggers the release of growth hormone, supporting tissue repair, muscle development and cellular regeneration.

Immunity – during sleep, the immune system produces and releases cytokines and antibodies to defend against pathogens.

The science of sleep

Sleep comprises alternating phases, each with distinct characteristics and functions. A full cycle lasts about 90 minutes, and we typically experience four to six cycles per night.

Non-REM sleep

The first three stages are non-REM sleep:

N1 (light sleep): a brief transition from wakefulness to slumber. Muscle activity slows and occasional twitches may occur.

N2 (light sleep): heart rate and breathing regularise, body temperature drops and the brain alternates between bursts of activity (sleep spindles) and quieter periods. Sleep spindles are thought to aid memory and learning. Around half of total sleep time is spent in N2.

N3 (deep sleep): also called slow-wave sleep, this is the most restorative phase. Blood pressure falls, breathing and heart rate reach their lowest levels, and growth hormone is secreted. Deep sleep typically accounts for 10–20% of the night.

(Some systems distinguish a fourth stage, N4, for even slower brain waves and greater restoration, though many merge it with N3.)

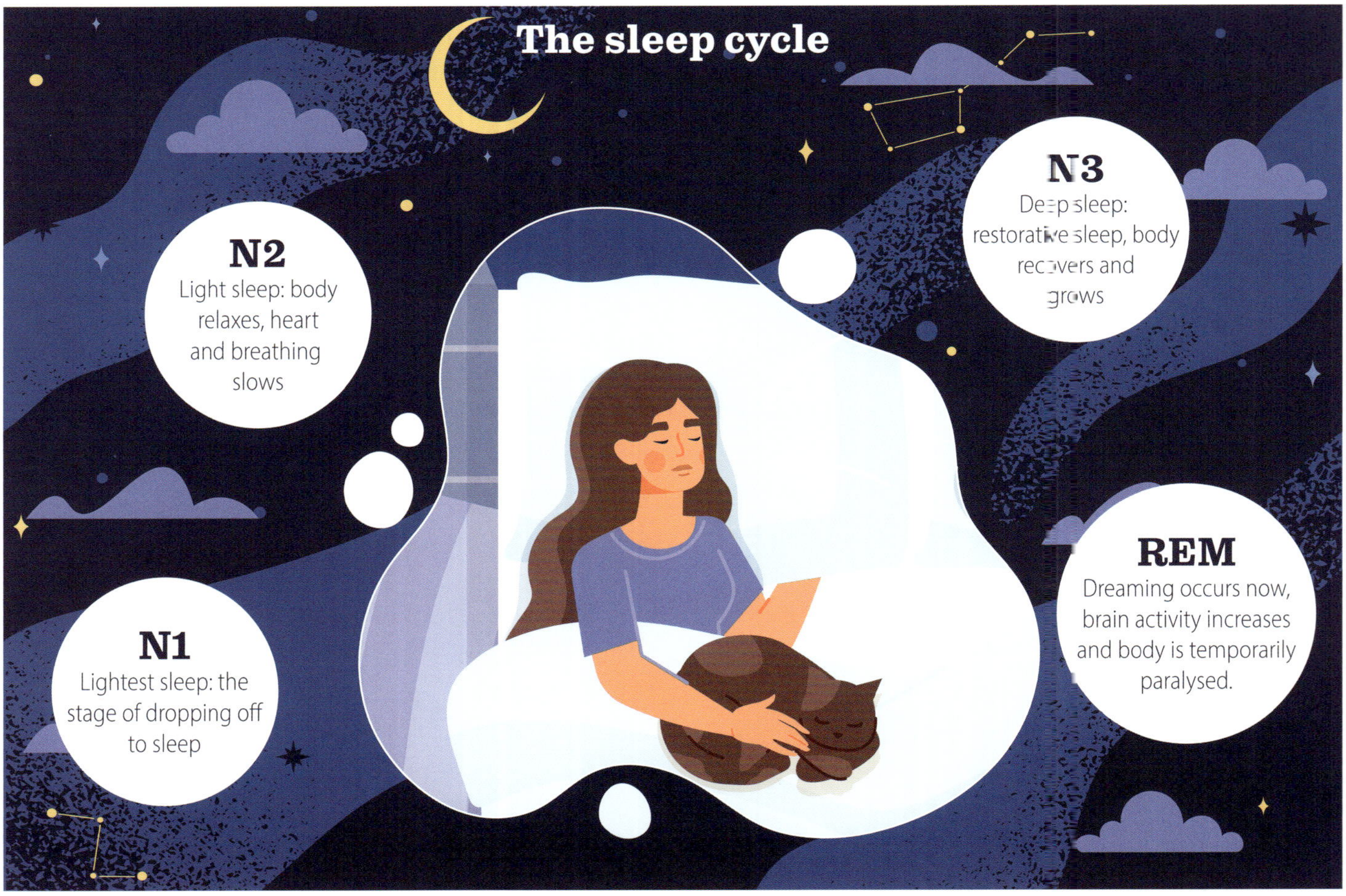

REM sleep

Next comes REM sleep when brain activity intensifies to resemble wakefulness and vivid dreams often occur. The body remains effectively paralysed to prevent us acting out our dreams. REM sleep usually makes up 20–25% of our total rest and lengthens towards morning, so early-morning sleep is often dominated by dream-filled cycles.

Circadian rhythms

Underlying our sleep-wake cycles is the circadian rhythm – an internal clock running on a roughly 24-hour cycle, directed by the brain's suprachiasmatic nucleus and influenced by environmental cues such as light and temperature. Exposure to natural daylight synchronises our rhythm, helping us feel alert by day and sleepy by night. Conversely, artificial light – especially blue light from screens – can delay sleep onset and diminish sleep quality.

Maintaining healthy sleep habits

Consistency is key to harnessing the full benefits of sleep. A regular sleep schedule – retiring and rising at the same time each day – reinforces your circadian rhythm. A restful environment free from noise, bright lights and electronic distractions promotes deep, uninterrupted sleep. Other helpful strategies include:

- limiting caffeine and alcohol, particularly in the afternoon and evening
- engaging in regular physical activity, but avoiding vigorous exercise close to bedtime
- practising relaxation techniques such as progressive muscle relaxation or meditation
- reserving the bed for sleep and sex only, strengthening the mental association between bedroom and slumber

By prioritising sleep hygiene, we maximise the restorative power of each night's rest.

The broader health implications of sleep

Beyond immediate performance and wellbeing, sleep exerts profound long-term effects on health. Chronic sleep debt is associated with increased risk of obesity, diabetes, cardiovascular disease and certain cancers. Inadequate sleep also impairs immune function, making infections more likely and recovery slower.

Mental health disorders such as depression and anxiety frequently co-occur with sleep disturbances. While insomnia can be a symptom of these conditions, evidence suggests that persistent sleep problems may also contribute to their onset. Addressing sleep issues early – through lifestyle adjustments or professional treatment – can play a pivotal role in preventing or alleviating mood disorders.

Sleep is far more than passive downtime. It is a vital, active process underpinning every aspect of our health and functioning – from memory consolidation and emotional resilience to tissue repair and immune defence. Given the serious consequences of sleep deprivation for individuals and society, we must recognise sleep as a cornerstone of wellbeing.

Armed with knowledge of sleep stages, circadian rhythms and the many functions sleep serves, we can take informed steps to optimise our nightly rest. The time we spend asleep is not wasted; it is an essential investment in our health, performance and happiness.

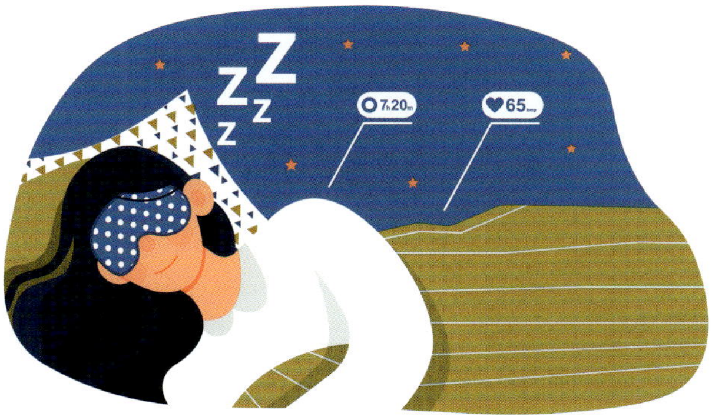

Complete a sleep diary

Grab a sheet of paper and divide it into four columns labelled 'Time I went to bed', 'Time I woke up', 'How I felt on waking', and 'Notes (dreams, disturbances)'.

Use the information from the article to predict what you might record in each column if you slept poorly one night.

Spend 5 minutes filling in your mock diary based on what you think your body and mind would experience after a night of inadequate sleep.

Design a sleep vocabulary crossword

Choose ten key terms from the article (for example 'circadian', 'spindles', 'REM', 'immunity').

Create clues for each term, some straightforward definitions, some more cryptic.

Draw or use an online tool to lay out a 10×10 crossword grid and fill in your words.

Swap with a classmate and solve each other's puzzles, then check your answers together.

Design a healthy-sleep poster

On an A3 sheet or poster-making paper, sketch at least five top tips for getting better sleep, drawing on the 'maintaining healthy sleep habits' section.

Include a mixture of text and illustrations – for example, a clock to show 'go to bed and wake at the same time' or an 'off' symbol over a smartphone to represent avoiding screens.

Add a catchy slogan (e.g., 'Power up with proper rest!') and decorate with colours and icons to make it engaging.

Be prepared to display your poster in the classroom.

The importance of sleep

We need time to dream!

Whether it's the longer lighter days, exam pressures, day-to-day adulting or other stressors, a good night of sleep can be very helpful in managing these stressors.

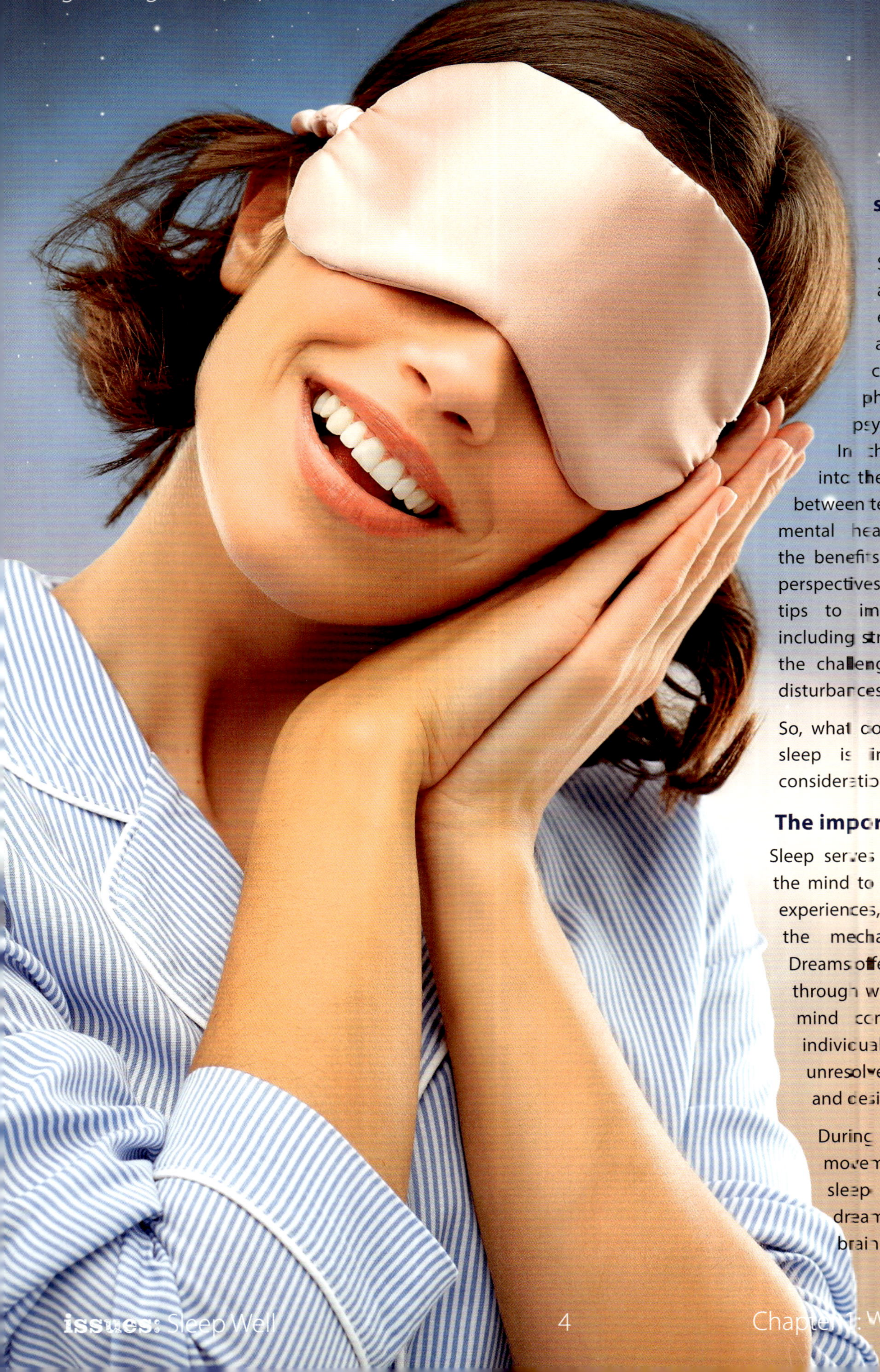

Understanding sleep and mental health

Sleep is a fundamental aspect of human life, especially during adolescence, a period characterised by rapid physical, emotional, and psychological changes. In this article, we delve into the intricate relationship between teen sleep patterns and mental health. While exploring the benefits of sleep from varied perspectives, we also offer practical tips to improve sleep quality, including strategies for navigating the challenges of summer sleep disturbances.

So, what do we think about why sleep is important? Well one consideration is…

The importance of dreams

Sleep serves as a crucial time for the mind to process and integrate experiences, particularly through the mechanism of dreaming. Dreams offer a symbolic language through which the subconscious mind communicates, allowing individuals to explore unresolved emotions, conflicts, and desires.

During the rapid eye movement (REM) stage of sleep which is when most dreaming occurs, the brain engages in intricate processes of memory consolidation and emotional regulation. Dreams provide a safe space for the mind to reenact and explore significant events or emotions that may be too overwhelming or complex to process consciously during waking hours.

When individuals experience disruptions in their sleep patterns, such as insomnia or insufficient sleep duration, the natural cycle of processing experiences through dreams may be compromised. As a result, unresolved emotions and conflicts may remain unprocessed or inadequately integrated into conscious awareness. This can lead to a build-up of emotional distress and contribute to declining mental health over time.

Therapeutically, addressing sleep disturbances involves not only restoring healthy sleep patterns but also exploring the underlying emotional and psychological factors that may be contributing to sleep difficulties. By encouraging clients to explore their dreams and the emotions they evoke, therapists can facilitate a deeper understanding of unconscious processes and help clients integrate their experiences more effectively.

In therapy, techniques such as dream analysis, journalling, and imagery rehearsal may be utilised to explore the symbolic language of dreams and uncover underlying conflicts or unresolved emotions. By bringing these unconscious processes into conscious awareness, clients can gain insight into their emotional landscape and work towards resolving internal conflicts, reducing emotional distress, and promoting overall mental wellbeing.

The importance of sleep:

From TMH's standpoint in the therapeutic field, sleep serves as a crucial time for the mind to process emotions, consolidate memories, and regulate mood. Adolescents, in particular, undergo significant emotional upheavals as they navigate identity formation and interpersonal relationships. Adequate sleep provides them with the necessary mental rest and rejuvenation to cope with these challenges effectively.

Physiologically, sleep plays a vital role in cognitive function, hormone regulation, and overall wellbeing. During sleep, the brain undergoes essential processes such as memory consolidation and neural repair. Disruptions in sleep patterns can impair cognitive abilities, increase stress hormone levels, and contribute to mental health struggles such as depression and anxiety.

Tips for improving sleep

1. Establish a consistent sleep schedule: Encourage teens to maintain a regular sleep-wake cycle, even on weekends, to regulate their internal body clock.

2. Create a relaxing bedtime routine: Incorporate calming activities such as reading, baths, or listening to soothing music to signal to the brain that it's time to wind down.

3. Limit screen time before bed: The blue light emitted by electronic devices can disrupt the production of melatonin, a hormone essential for sleep. Encourage teens to avoid screens at least an hour before bedtime.

4. Create a comfortable sleep environment: Ensure the bedroom is conducive to sleep by keeping it cool, dark, and quiet. Invest in a comfortable mattress and pillows to promote restful sleep.

5. Practice stress reduction techniques: Teach teens relaxation techniques such as certain breathing exercises to slow down breathing, or mindfulness meditation to alleviate anxiety and promote relaxation before bedtime.

Dealing with summer sleep challenges

The longer daylight hours and warmer temperatures during summer can pose additional challenges to maintaining healthy sleep habits. Here are some tips to address summer sleep disturbances:

1. Use blackout curtains: Install blackout curtains to block out excess sunlight, creating a darker environment conducive to sleep.

2. Stay cool: Use fans or air conditioning to regulate bedroom temperature, ensuring a comfortable sleep environment.

3. Adjust bedtime routine: Encourage teens to adjust their bedtime routine to account for the extended daylight hours. Dimming lights and engaging in relaxing activities can help signal to the body that it's time to sleep despite the brighter evenings.

4. Practice good sleep hygiene: Reinforce the importance of maintaining consistent sleep habits, even during the summer months, to mitigate the effects of seasonal disruptions.

Understanding the relationship between teen sleep patterns and mental health is crucial for promoting overall wellbeing during adolescence. Especially when we consider at the time of writing, many adolescents are preparing or going through exams for GCSE/A-levels.

By integrating psychological and physiological aspects of sleep, we can appreciate the multifaceted benefits of sleep. By implementing practical tips for improving sleep quality and addressing seasonal challenges, teens can enhance their mental health and thrive during this transformative stage of life.

1 May 2024

The above information is reprinted with kind permission from Teenage Mental Health.
© 2025 Teenage Mental Health

www.teenagementalhealth.co.uk

Why do we usually sleep at night? What happens when we don't sleep? Expert insights into this essential part of our lives

An article by The Conversation.

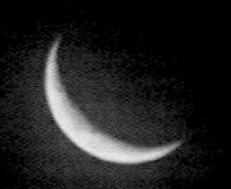

By Karine Scheuermaier, Associate Professor in Physiology, Chair of Science Committee, South African Society for Sleep and Health, Member of the World Sleep Society, University of the Witwatersrand; Alison Bentley, Honorary Lecturer in Family Medicine, University of the Witwatersrand; Dale Rae, Director of Sleep Science and Associate Professor at the Faculty of Health Sciences, University of Cape Town; Francesco Xavier Gomez-Olive Casas, Research Manager at MRC/Wits Agincourt Research Unit, University of the Witwatersrand; Gosia Lipinska, Associate Professor, University of Cape Town, Jonathan Davy, Senior lecturer, Rhodes University; Joshua Davimes, Senior Lecturer in Anatomical Sciences, University of the Witwatersrand; Nomathemba Chandiwana, Principal Scientist at Ezintsha, University of the Witwatersrand; & Oluwatosin Olorunmoteni, Neurodevelopmental Paediatrician, Obafemi Awolowo University

Sleep is as essential to our health as food and water. It is important to a number of brain functions, including how nerve cells communicate with each other. We sleep for a third of our lives and there are many restorative processes going on during sleep that are needed to stay healthy.

Why do we usually sleep at night? What happens when we don't sleep? On World Sleep Day, Nadine Dreyer asks a group of experts to tell us more about this essential part of our lives.

Why do we need sleep and why do we sleep better at night?

We sleep for a third of our lives, yet it is only when we cannot sleep or when we experience poor quality sleep that we really start noticing it.

During sleep, our muscle activity drops, our breathing slows down, and our heart rate and blood pressure decrease. At the same time our brain actively clears toxins, which cause neurodegenerative diseases.

It also consolidates memories, wiping out 'useless' ones during deep sleep, known as slow wave sleep.

All this allows us to start afresh the following day.

Our lives are organised around our sleep-wake schedule. As we're a diurnal species, our master clock in the brain, which maintains many of our 24-hour rhythms, schedules our period of activity with daylight, and our period of rest with the night.

In some other animals, like rodents, evolutionary pressure has pushed those species to become nocturnal, which allows them to scurry and feed outside the view of their diurnal (daytime) or crepuscular (twilight) predators.

Not sleeping at the right time has been associated with poor health. Some of the side-effects are poorer cognitive performance, lower energy and worse mental health.

There's also a higher risk of developing neurodegenerative diseases such as Alzheimer's and a higher risk of developing high blood pressure and diabetes.

After a poor night's sleep, we try to get on with our lives but research has shown this is not so easy. During the COVID-19 pandemic and the strictest lockdown, South Africans rated their sleep quality as poorer, with more insomnia symptoms. These were both in turn associated with worse levels of depression and anxiety.

What happens when we don't sleep?

Sleep is a state of vulnerability where a 'rest and digest' state dominates over the 'fight and flight' state when we are awake.

Our early sleep 'scans' the environment before allowing us to dive into deeper stages of sleep.

When a rupture in this consolidated bout of sleep happens, we will start complaining 'I haven't slept enough' or 'I slept really badly last night'.

Such ruptures include those induced by specific sleep disorders like sleep apnoea or insomnia.

Sleep apnoea leads to unconscious sleep interruptions due to upper airways obstruction and can lead to hypertension and increased risk of diabetes.

Research in rural Mpumalanga province in South Africa found one out of three older adults had moderate to severe sleep apnoea and this was associated with a higher risk of cardiovascular disease. Yet there is no treatment in the public health system for this common sleep disorder.

Certain situations disrupt sleep: parents tending to their young children, doctors being awake while on call, loud generator noises during night-time electricity cuts, mosquitoes, or worse, gunshots or sounds of violence waking us up from our slumber, signalling danger.

Sleep health inequity in South Africa is also driven by socioeconomic status.

A recent study on sleep in men and women living in the urban township of Khayelitsha in South Africa's Western Cape province showed that poor sleep quality was associated with fear of falling asleep in a violent environment. Sleep was disturbed by strange noises, fear of attacks and dreams about past traumatic experiences.

Electronic devices make it difficult to sleep. Why?

Even though our biology is meant to make us sleep at night, several societal, technological changes have progressively decreased our sleep opportunity.

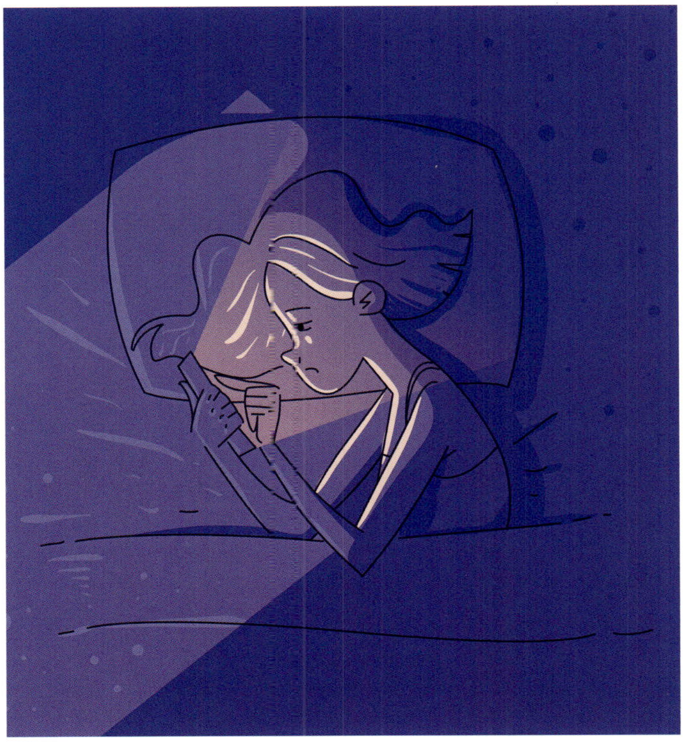

Our sleep timing is controlled by our master circadian clock. This clock is exquisitely sensitive to light, so exposure to bright light and blue light such as that emitted from electronic devices such as smartphones shifts our bedtime to a later time.

In our recently published study of adolescent sleep in Nigeria, adolescents in urban areas slept less and sleep quality was worse.

Sleep duration was shorter, due to bedtimes being later but waking times in the morning similar to those of adolescents in rural areas. The use of electronic devices at night by urban Nigerian adolescents was associated with shorter sleep duration.

This is one example of a growing body of research that highlights the negative consequences of nocturnal tech use on sleep, even in African societies.

What are key habits to help people sleep better?

The most important habit is to take sleep as seriously as a healthy diet and regular exercise.

We advise the following:

- Keep regular wake times and bedtimes. This helps us sleep at the best time with respect to our master clock's rhythm. This in turn helps ensure a consolidated bout of sleep.
- Aim for an average of 7 to 9 hours of sleep each night.
- Avoid watching screens one hour before normal bedtime. If this is unavoidable, choose the lowest brightness and add the orange night screen setting. Rather read a book under a bedside light.
- Get outdoor light during the day to strengthen the master clock's circadian (near 24-hour) rhythm.
- Do some form of physical activity once a day. This helps build sleep pressure and also strengthens the master clock's rhythms.
- Avoid alcohol before bedtime as this is associated with disrupted sleep.
- Avoid caffeine and stimulants after noon.
- Try to sleep in a quiet, cool and dark or dimly lit environment.

14 March 2024

THE CONVERSATION

The above information is reprinted with kind permission from The Conversation.

© 2010-2025, The Conversation Trust (UK) Limited

www.theconversation.com

How much sleep do we need?

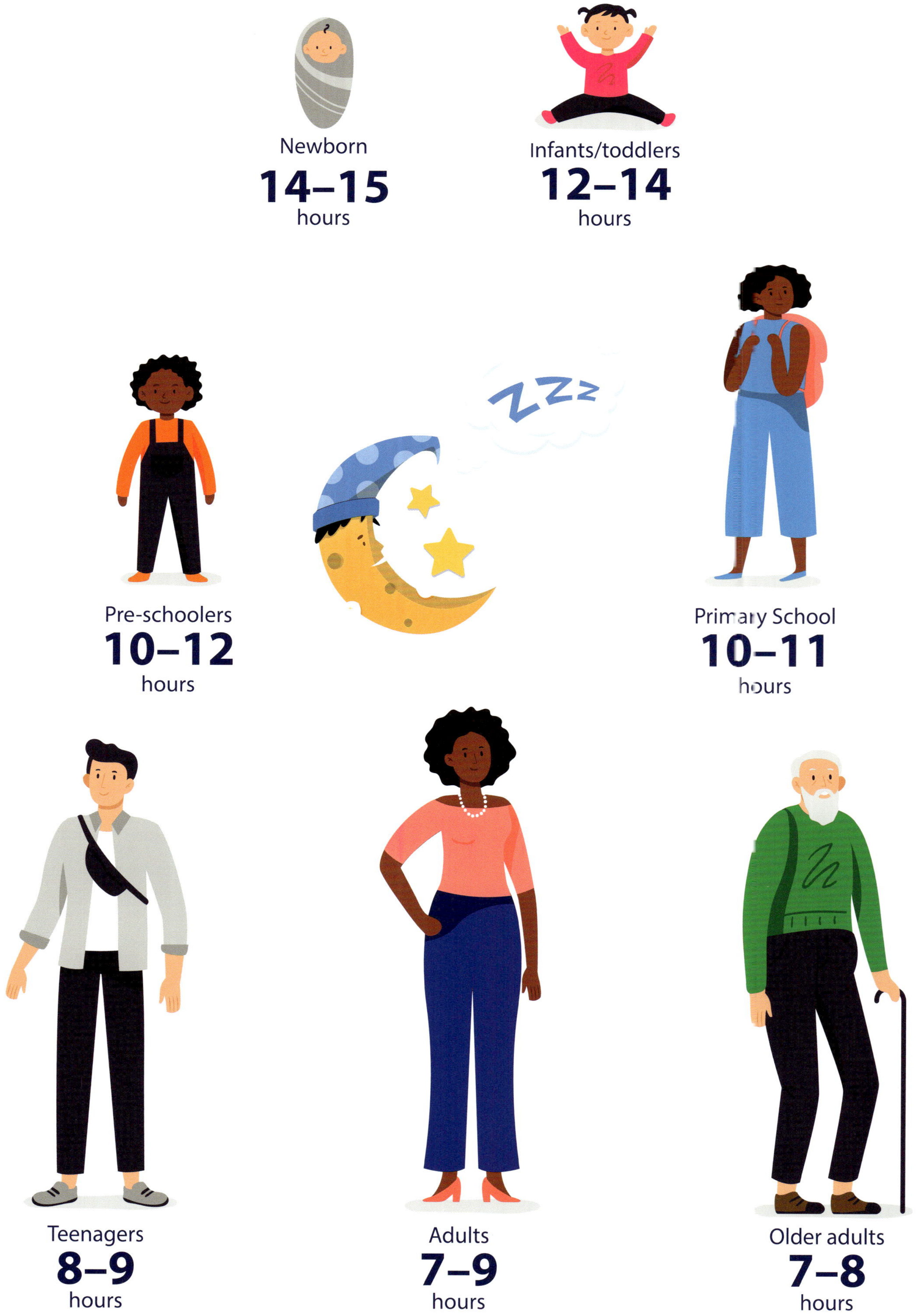

Five sleep myths busted

By Kathryn Pinkham

After working with poor sleepers for over 13 years now, I've noticed more than a few sleep myths which crop up time and time again! From the amount of sleep we need, to whether or not caffeine will stop you sleeping, I thought I'd address some of these on my blog to help separate fact from fiction.

1. We all need eight hours of sleep

Probably the most common sleep myth out there, the magical eight hours of sleep! The truth is, everyone's sleep needs are different, and quality is more important than quantity. In fact, it's the quality of sleep you get that matters rather than the quantity. The best way to do this is by slightly restricting your time in bed, so you have a higher sleep drive and are more likely to fall asleep quicker, and more deeply. So if you aren't getting eight hours every night, don't worry, as long as your sleep is good quality.

2. Sleeping pills aren't addictive

As a short-term solution, sleeping pills can be very effective. However, over time they tend to stop working as well, so we have to take a higher dose in order to get the same results. This can lead to something called rebound insomnia, meaning that on nights when you take a pill you actually end up sleeping even worse than before, leading to increased anxiety and further reliance on the medication. So, in the long term, they can become addictive both physically and psychologically. The best way to manage this is to use CBT techniques alongside medication, so over time you can safely wean yourself off.

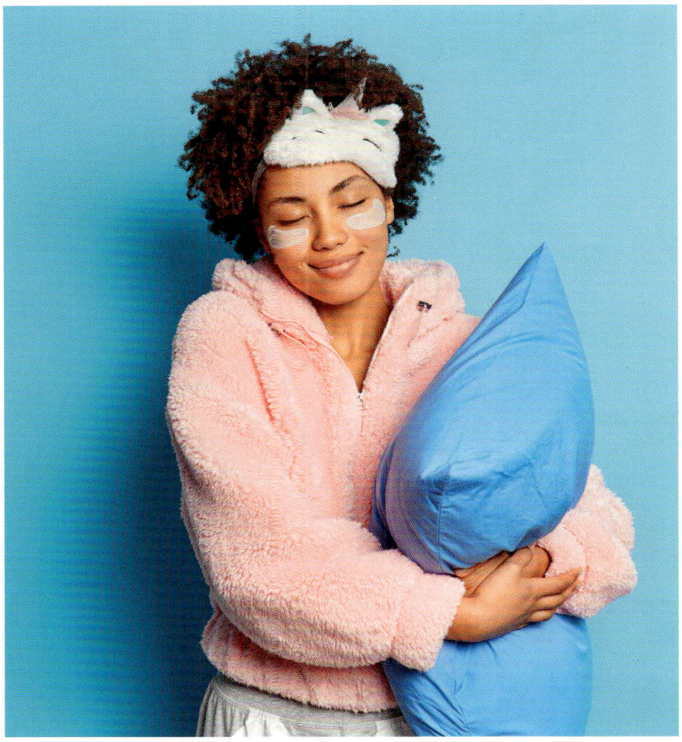

3. You have to be relaxed to sleep

Learning to relax is great, for both our physical and mental health. However, it is not true that the only reason you can't sleep is because you are not relaxed. In fact, if you try too hard to relax in order to sleep well, you can end up becoming hyper vigilant about sleep, resulting in worse sleep. Spend some time in the day learning to find ways that make you feel relaxed, such as exercise and mindfulness, but please remember that you don't need long and lengthy wind-down routines at bedtime in order to sleep. Spend your evenings doing things you enjoy rather than 'trying' to relax, and this way you are less likely to be over focused on sleep!

4. Caffeine is bad for your sleep

Caffeine is often regarded as the reason people can't sleep, and of course if you're drinking it straight before bed this could be the case; however, having a cup of tea or coffee in

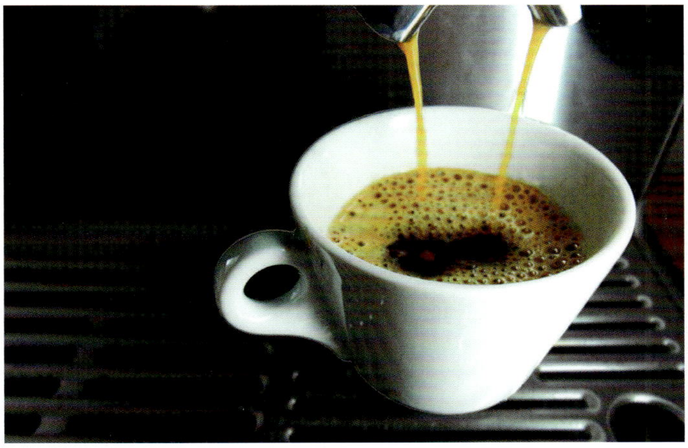

the morning, or one after your lunch, is unlikely to have a real impact on your sleep. So, if you love your tea or coffee, don't restrict yourself! Simply try not to drink later in the day, but if you feel tired in the morning or afternoon and need a little boost, then go ahead.

5. If you feel tired in the day, your sleep is to blame

Daytime sleepiness isn't always down to poor sleep. If you feel you sleep well, but are always feeling tired, then take a look at your stress levels. Time and time again I remind people that you can't out sleep a stressful life. Being in fight or flight mode leaves us feeling exhausted, so no amount of sleep will give you energy if you are mentally stressed.

12 October 2024

The above information is reprinted with kind permission from The Insomnia Clinic.
© 2025 The Insomnia Clinic

www.theinsomniaclinic.co.uk

Effects of lack of sleep on the body

Trouble with thinking and concentration

When you're tired, your focus, creativity and problem-solving skills suffer.

Memory issues

During sleep your brain builds connections that help you learn and remember things. Not getting enough sleep harms both short-term and long-term memory.

Risk of diabetes

Sleep loss disrupts how your body uses insulin, the hormone that lowers blood sugar. As a result, you may have higher blood sugar levels and a greater chance of developing type 2 diabetes.

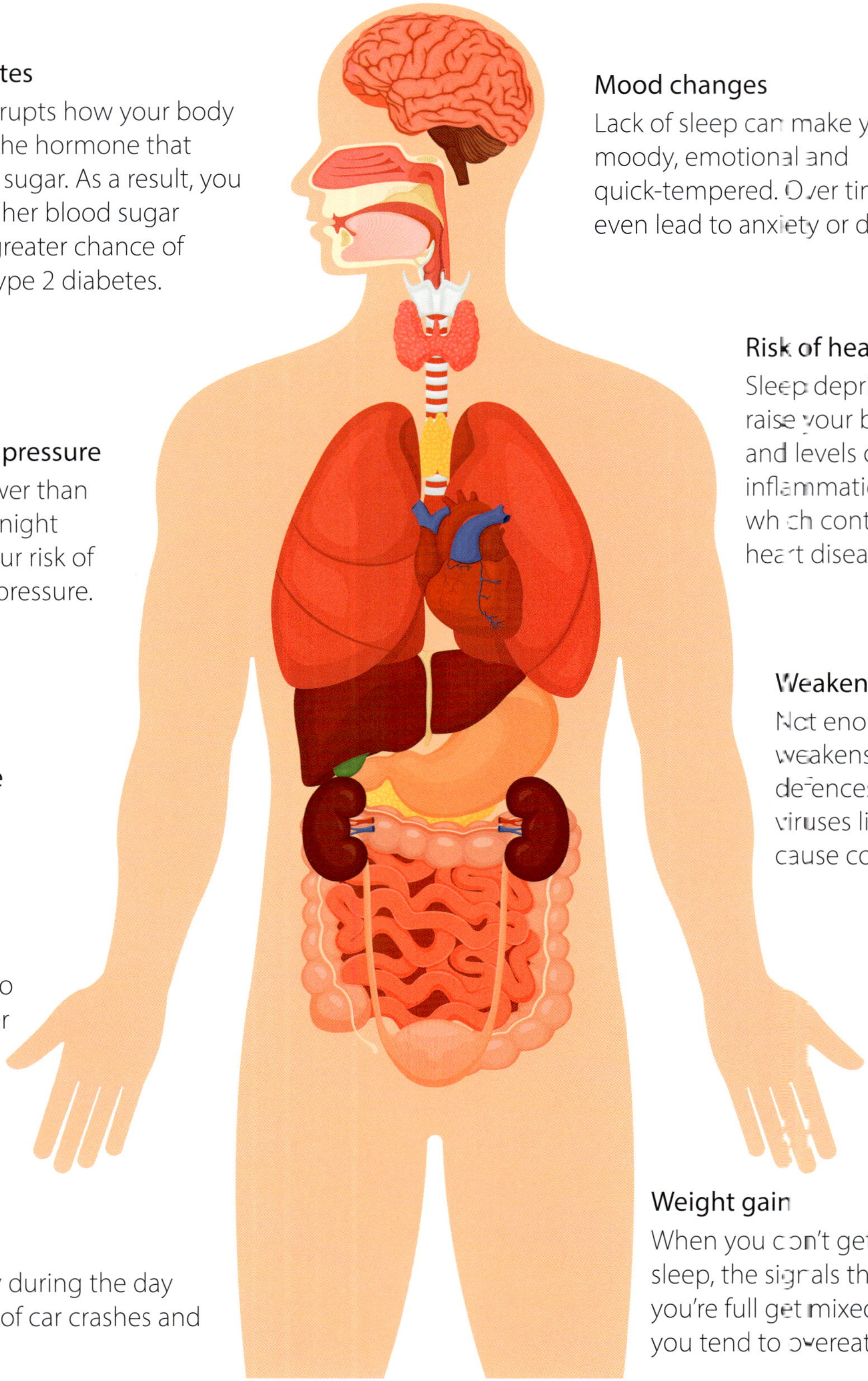

Mood changes

Lack of sleep can make you moody, emotional and quick-tempered. Over time it may even lead to anxiety or depression.

Risk of heart disease

Sleep deprivation can raise your blood pressure and levels of inflammation, both of which contribute to heart disease.

High blood pressure

Sleeping fewer than five hours a night increases your risk of high blood pressure.

Weakened immunity

Not enough sleep weakens your body's defences against viruses like those that cause colds and flu.

Poor balance

Being sleepy affects your coordination and balance, making you more prone to falls and other accidents.

Weight gain

When you can't get enough sleep, the signals that tell you you're full get mixed up – so you tend to overeat.

Accidents

Feeling drowsy during the day raises your risk of car crashes and other mishaps.

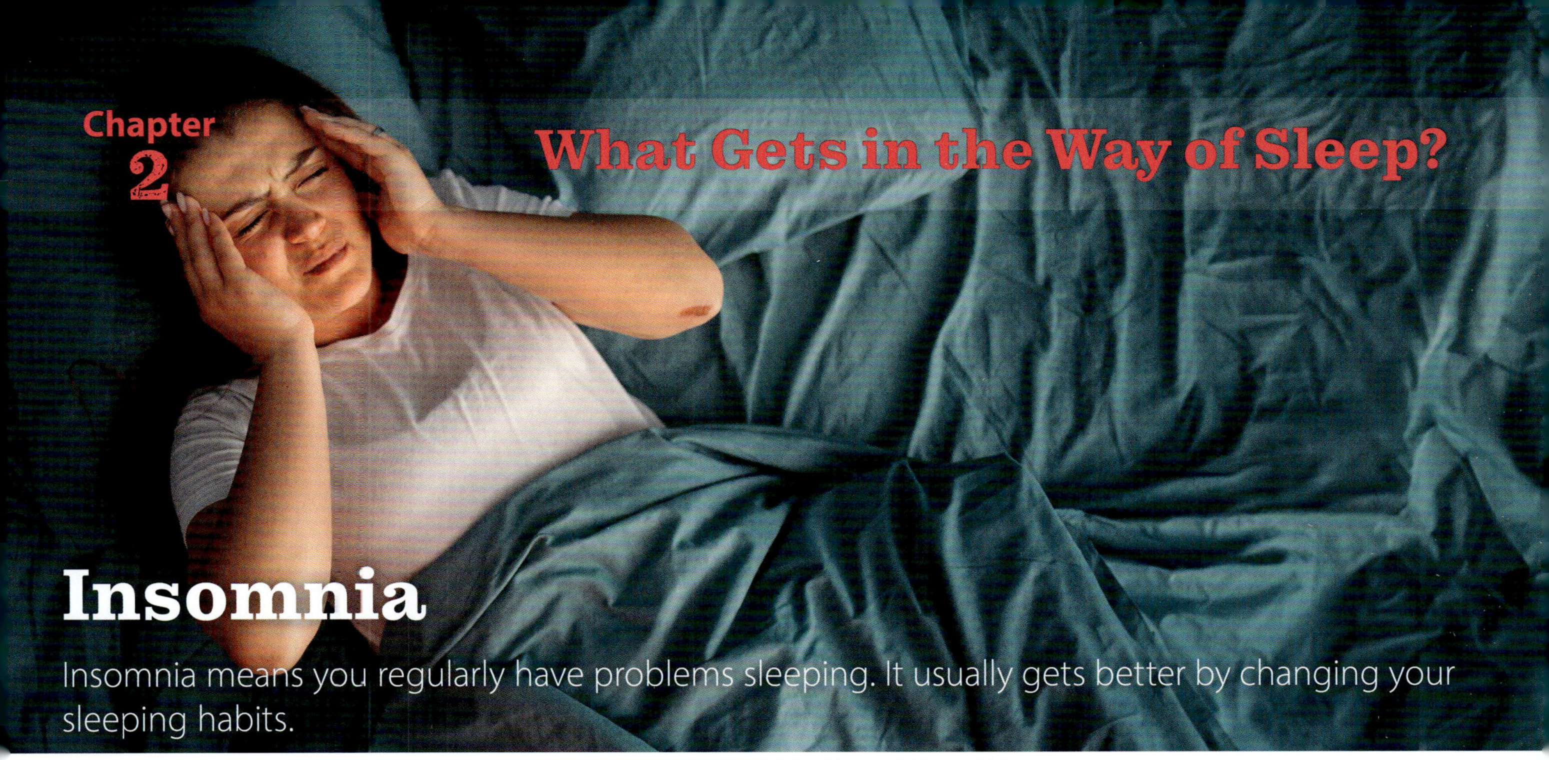

Chapter 2

What Gets in the Way of Sleep?

Insomnia

Insomnia means you regularly have problems sleeping. It usually gets better by changing your sleeping habits.

Symptoms of insomnia

You have insomnia if you regularly:

- find it hard to go to sleep
- wake up several times during the night
- lie awake at night
- wake up early and cannot go back to sleep
- still feel tired after waking up
- find it hard to nap during the day even though you're tired
- feel tired and irritable during the day
- find it difficult to concentrate during the day because you're tired

If you have insomnia for a short time (less than 3 months) it's called short-term insomnia. Insomnia that lasts 3 months or longer is called long-term insomnia.

How much sleep you need

Everyone needs different amounts of sleep.

On average:

- adults need 7 to 9 hours
- children need 9 to 13 hours
- toddlers and babies need 12 to 17 hours

You probably do not get enough sleep if you're constantly tired during the day.

What causes insomnia

The most common causes of insomnia are:

- stress, anxiety or depression
- noise
- a room that's too hot or cold
- uncomfortable beds
- alcohol, caffeine or nicotine
- illegal drugs like cocaine or ecstasy
- jet lag
- shift work

How you can treat insomnia yourself

Insomnia usually gets better by changing your sleeping habits.

Do

- ✔ go to bed and wake up at the same time every day
- ✔ relax at least 1 hour before bed, for example, take a bath or read a book
- ✔ make sure your bedroom is dark and quiet – use curtains, blinds, an eye mask or ear plugs if needed
- ✔ exercise regularly during the day
- ✔ make sure your mattress, pillows and covers are comfortable

Don't

- ✘ do not smoke or drink alcohol, tea or coffee at least 6 hours before going to bed
- ✘ do not eat a big meal late at night
- ✘ do not exercise at least 4 hours before bed
- ✘ do not watch television or use devices, like smartphones, right before going to bed, because the blue light makes you more awake
- ✘ do not nap during the day
- ✘ do not drive when you feel sleepy
- ✘ do not sleep in after a bad night's sleep and stick to your regular sleeping hours instead

19 March 2024

The above information is reprinted with kind permission from the NHS.

© Crown Copyright 2025

This information is licensed under the Open Government Licence v3.0

To view this licence, visit http://www.nationalarchives.gov.uk/doc/open-government-licence/

OGL

www.nhs.uk

10 Reasons why you can't sleep

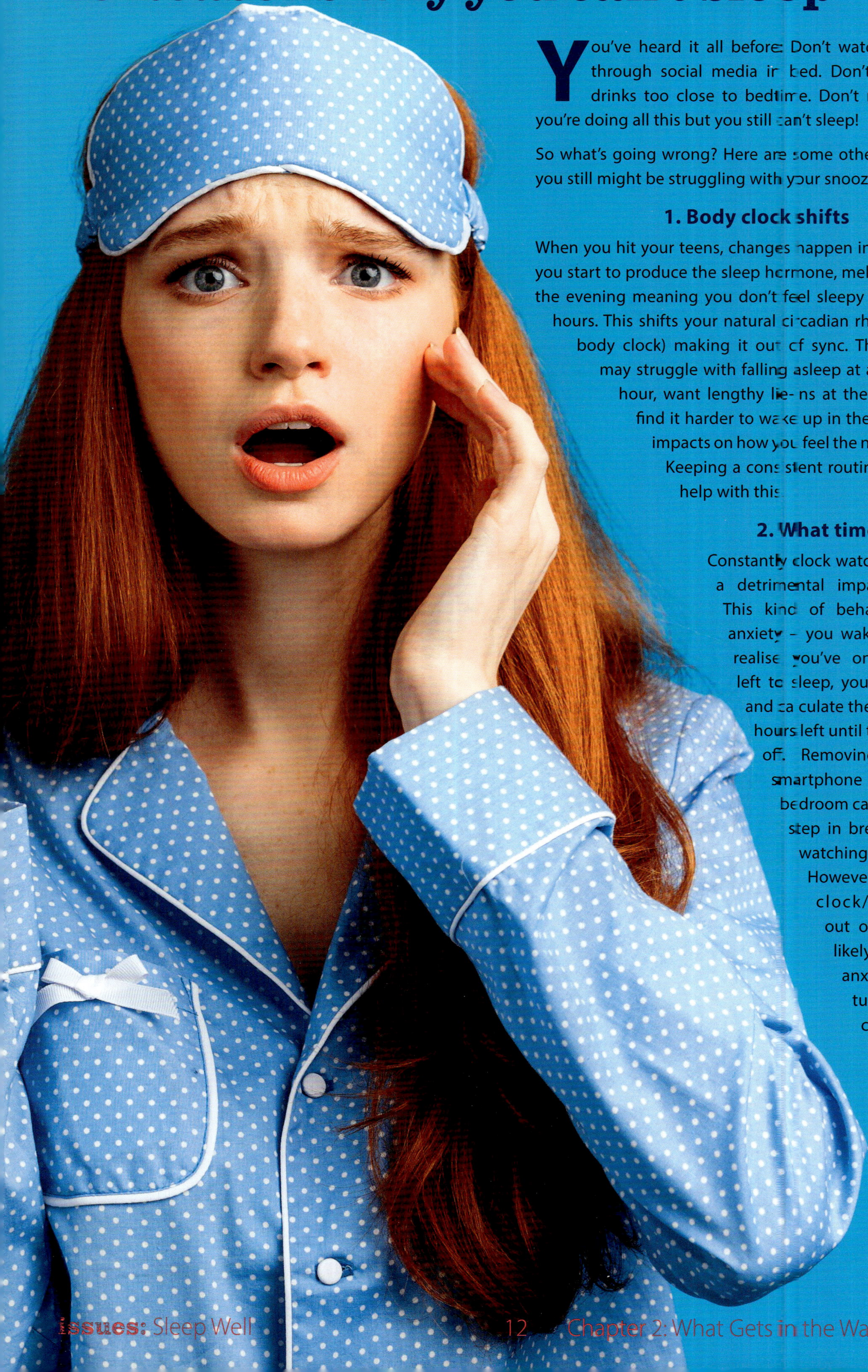

You've heard it all before: Don't watch TV or scroll through social media in bed. Don't drink energy drinks too close to bedtime. Don't nap... and yet you're doing all this but you still can't sleep!

So what's going wrong? Here are some other reasons why you still might be struggling with your snoozing.

1. Body clock shifts

When you hit your teens, changes happen in the brain and you start to produce the sleep hormone, melatonin, later in the evening meaning you don't feel sleepy until the early hours. This shifts your natural circadian rhythm (internal body clock) making it out of sync. This means you may struggle with falling asleep at an appropriate hour, want lengthy lie-ins at the weekend and find it harder to wake up in the morning. This impacts on how you feel the next day – tired! Keeping a consistent routine in place will help with this.

2. What time is it

Constantly clock watching can have a detrimental impact on sleep. This kind of behaviour creates anxiety – you wake at 2am and realise you've only five hours left to sleep, you wake at 4am and calculate there's only three hours left until the alarm goes off. Removing the clock/smartphone from the bedroom can be a positive step in breaking a clock watching routine. However if having the clock/smartphone out of the room is likely to make you anxious, why not turn it around or cover it.

3. Feeling overwhelmed

Whether it's worries over schoolwork, friendships, relationships, growing up, feeling anxious in bed leads to difficulty in falling asleep and staying asleep. The first step is to write down any worries, or even your homework to-do list, before you go to bed as it helps to clear the mind. There are some really nice journals out there that you can use. Talk to someone you feel comfortable with – a friend, parent, family member or teacher – as it can help put worries into perspective. There are organisations such as Young Minds who can also help.

4. Hunger pangs

While we don't recommend eating a big meal before bedtime, some people do find a small bedtime snack helpful. If you go to bed hungry, you're likely to wake up with hunger pangs. A great bedtime snack could be oatcakes and cheese, nut butter on wholemeal toast or a small bowl of low sugar cereal.

5. Light

Street lights, TV standby button, notification light on your smartphone and even digital alarm clocks could all be a factor in keeping you awake. Make sure you're using blackout blinds or heavy lined curtains to block out outside light. Switch off the TV at the mains and don't be tempted to charge your mobile phone in the bedroom. Even this small amount of light disrupts your internal body clock and decreases your melatonin production, making you feel less sleepy.

6. Your bed is too old/uncomfortable

Everyone loves their bed, don't they? If you don't, maybe it's time for a new one! Don't be afraid to speak to your parents if you find your current mattress is lumpy and bumpy. They don't sleep on it so they won't know if it's past its best or you've outgrown it.

7. Lazy lie-ins

Trying to make up for lack of sleep with extra time in bed at the weekend throws off your internal body clock. Where possible try to keep to a regular bed time and wake up time. Our bodies (and minds) thrive on routine.

8. Too much to do

Are you finding yourself scrimping on sleep because there's not enough time in the evening to get things done, such as hobbies, sporting activities and homework? Leaving no time to wind down makes falling asleep even harder. Remember you will think more clearly, be more focused and patient if you've had a good night's sleep.

9. Messy bedroom

A cluttered bedroom makes for a cluttered mind. You may not be able to make the bedroom a complete clutter-free zone but try to keep it as tidy as possible. Put clothes away, dirty cups in the dishwasher and tidy your working area. Although you sleep with your eyes closed – and can't see the clutter when you're asleep – it's the last thing you look at before you catch some ZZZs, which may influence any anxious or worrying thoughts.

10. Lack of routine

Having a bedtime routine isn't just for kids! If you are having trouble sleeping well, putting a sleep plan in place is the first step to getting sleep back on track. A routine prepares you for rest so it's important that you map out time to wind down in the evening before bed. A sleep routine should ideally last around an hour each night. Doing the same thing, at the same time, before bed each evening can help to strengthen your circadian rhythm and help you feel sleepy. Try some calm quiet activities to help you to relax and unwind – that could be drawing, puzzles, listening to music or reading. Avoid screens – they're visually stimulating and will decrease the production of the sleep hormone melatonin.

The above information is reprinted with kind permission from The Sleep Charity.
© 2025 The Sleep Charity

www.thesleepcharity.org.uk

Audit your bedroom environment

In pairs – take five minutes to walk around your own or a mock-up bedroom in the classroom.

List every source of light you can find (e.g., street-light through the window, TV standby, phone charger LED, digital clock).

For each, note how you could remove or reduce that light (e.g., blackout blinds, turning the TV off at the mains, covering the clock display).

Share your ideas with another pair and compare which solutions would be easiest to put in place.

Create a personal sleep plan poster

In small groups – choose one of the ten reasons for poor sleep (e.g., body-clock shifts, lack of routine, feeling overwhelmed).

On a poster, illustrate the problem and suggest three practical steps to fix it (e.g., 'write worries in a journal before bed' for feeling overwhelmed).

Use images, bullet points and a clear title so your poster can teach others in the class.

Sleeping patterns

By Milan Dinic

More Britons say they are night owls (44%) than early risers (33%).

Younger Britons are more likely to fall in the 'night owl' category than older generations: 51–59% of 16- to 39-year-olds say they are 'night owls', compared to 37–40% of those older than 40.

Seven out of 10 Britons (71%) say they always or usually go to bed at the same time every night, while 27% go to bed at different times each night.

Britons aged 16–24 (39%) are more likely than those aged 25–59 (28%) and those aged 60 and over (20%) to report going to bed at different times.

Britons tend to identify with being a night owl more than being an early riser

Are you more of an early riser or a night owl? %

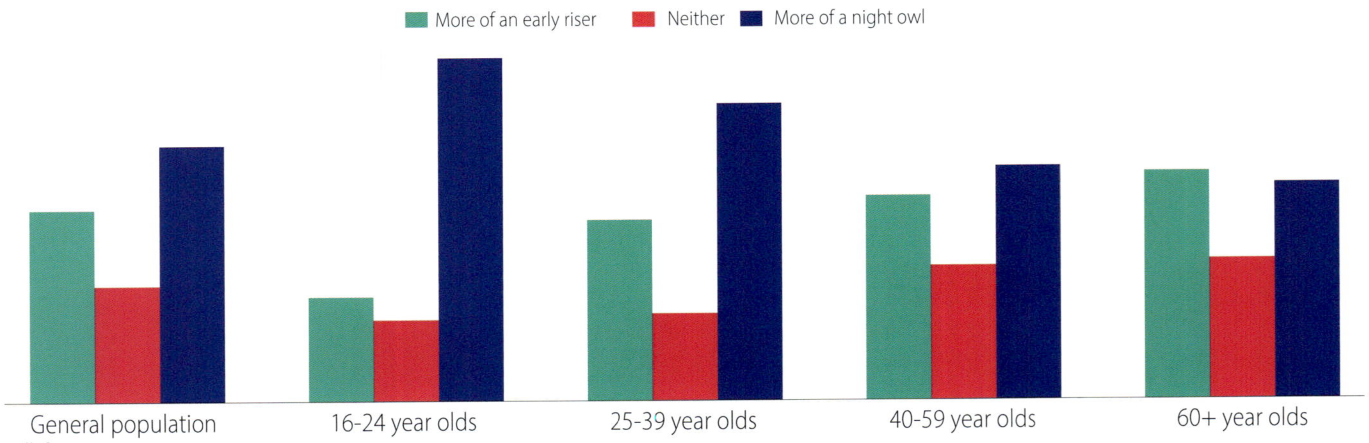

Source: YouGov

Around a quarter of Britons say they always or usually go to bed at different times every night

In terms of when you go to bed at night, which applies to you more…? %

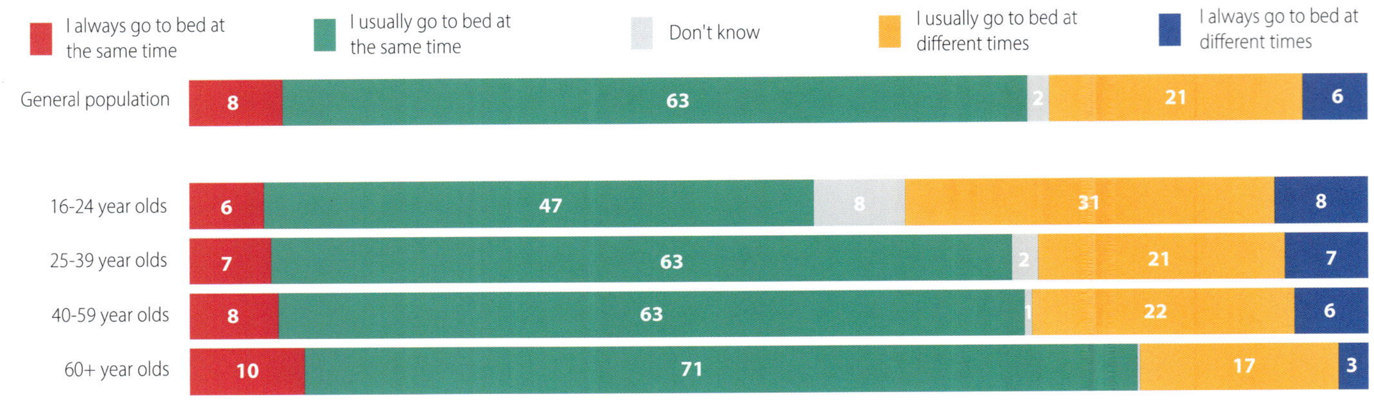

Source: YouGov

One in eight Britons, and a quarter of young people, say they go to bed after midnight

What time, on average, do you go to bed at night? %

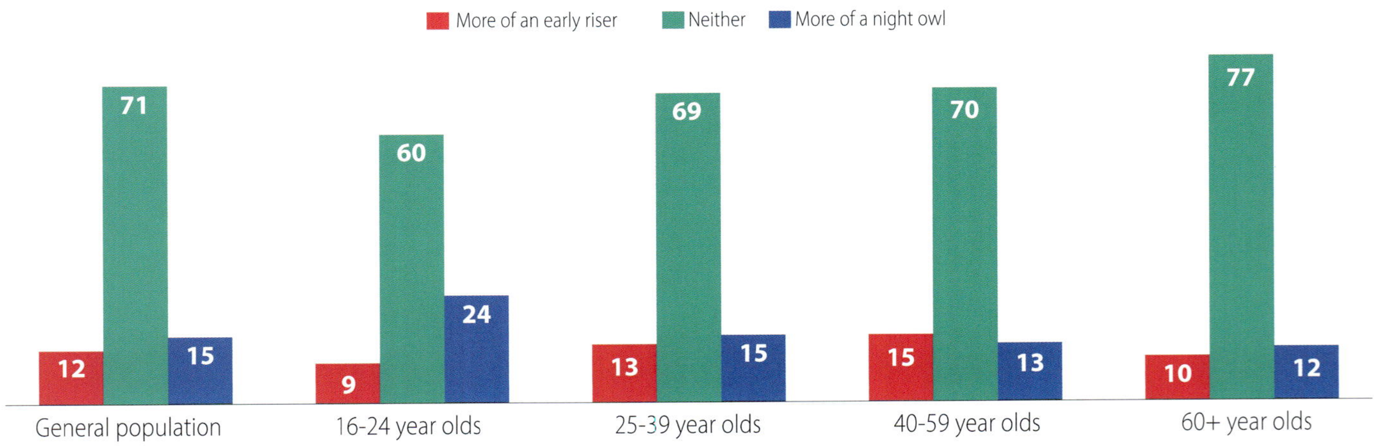

Source: YouGov

Early risers (85%) are significantly more likely to say they hit the sack at a regular time, compared to 60% of those who describe themselves as night owls.

About half of Britons (48%) go to sleep from around 10pm to around 11pm, while one in eight (12%) go to bed at around 9.30pm or earlier. Just over one in four (27%) go to bed between around 11:30pm and around 12.30am, while 11% of Britons turn in at around 1am or later.

Men are more likely than women to go to bed later at night: 43% of men go to bed from around 11:30pm onwards compared to 32% of women.

Younger Britons are the most likely to go to bed very late (at around 1am or later): 17% of 16–24 year olds say they do so, compared to 12% of those 25–39 and 8–9% of those aged 40 and above.

Women (20%) are more likely than men (14%) to take around an hour or longer to fall asleep.

One in eight Britons (13%) have fewer than six hours of sleep per night. The most common average sleep period is seven hours a night, which 35% of Britons say they get. One in five (22%) say they typically get six hours of sleep a night, while a similar number say they get eight hours a night (20%). Only 5% get nine hours of sleep or more, on average.

Half of Britons (49%) think they do not get enough sleep per night, with this applying more to women (53%) than men (45%).

Those aged 60 and older (51%) are more likely than everyone else (35–38%) to be satisfied with the amount of sleep they get.

Women aged 25–59 are substantially more likely than other age groups to say they don't get enough sleep, at 58–60%.

Early risers are more likely than night owls to say they get enough sleep each night: 50% vs 37%.

Nine in ten (89%) Britons say their life would be improved if they had more sleep. Half (53%) said their life would improve 'very much' while a third (36%) said it would improve 'somewhat'.

Among Britons who think they do not get enough sleep, 59% say their life would be improved 'very much' and 34% say it would improve 'somewhat' if they had more shut-eye.

One in five Britons (20%) say they often have naps during the day, while 43% have them sometimes. A third of Britons (35%) never nap during the day.

Britons aged 60 and above are the most likely to take naps during the day, at 27%.

Daytime naps are more popular among Britons who sleep five hours a night or less (33%), compared to those who get six hours of sleep or more (16–23%).

Among Britons who ever nap, one in five (19%) think the perfect nap should be between 15 and 20 minutes, while a quarter (24%) say it should last between 20 and 30 minutes.

One in seven Britons say it only takes them five minutes to fall asleep

How long, on average, does it take you to get to sleep? %

Source: YouGov

One in eight Britons sleep for fewer than six hours a night

How many hours of sleep do you get, on average, a night? %

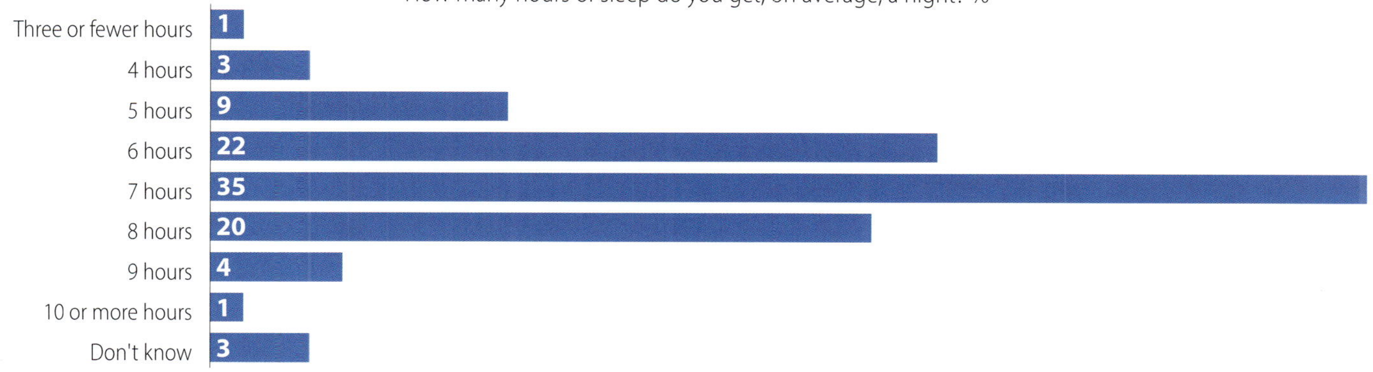

Source: YouGov

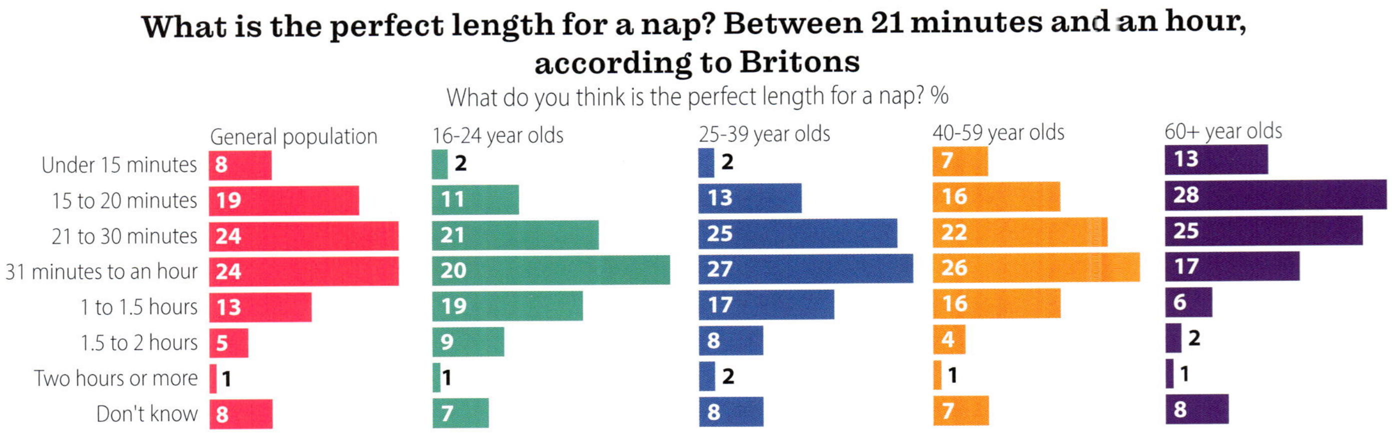

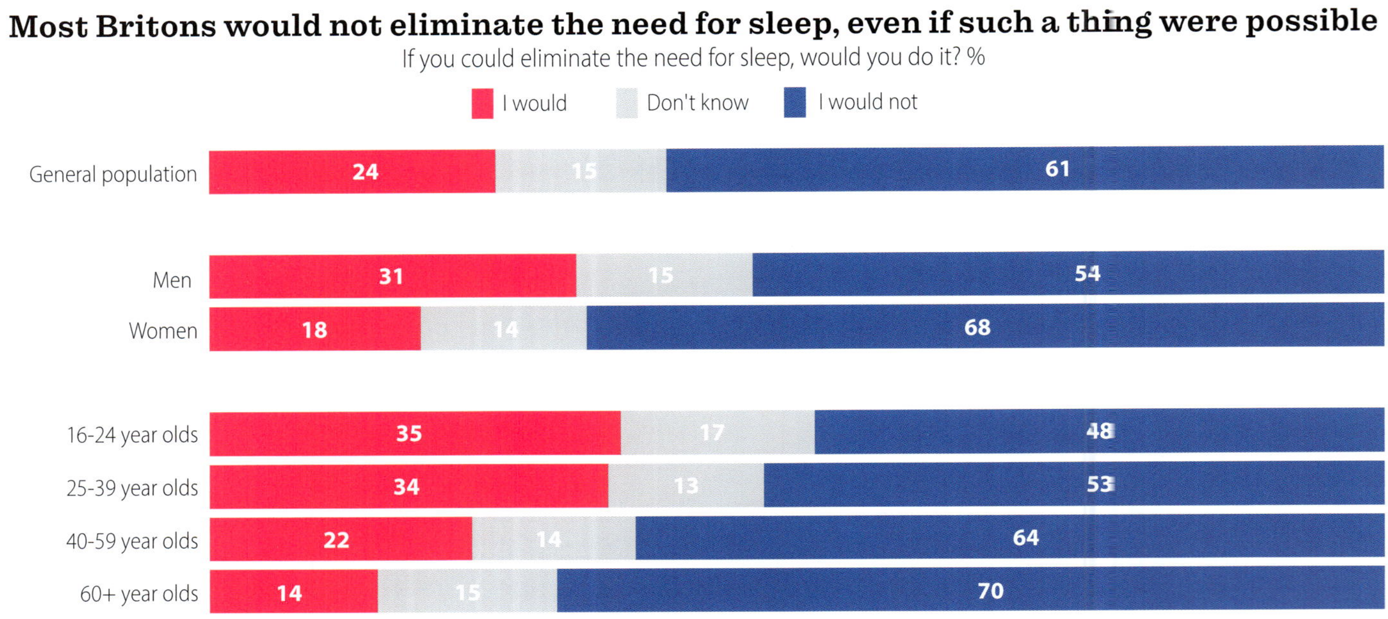

Source: YouGov

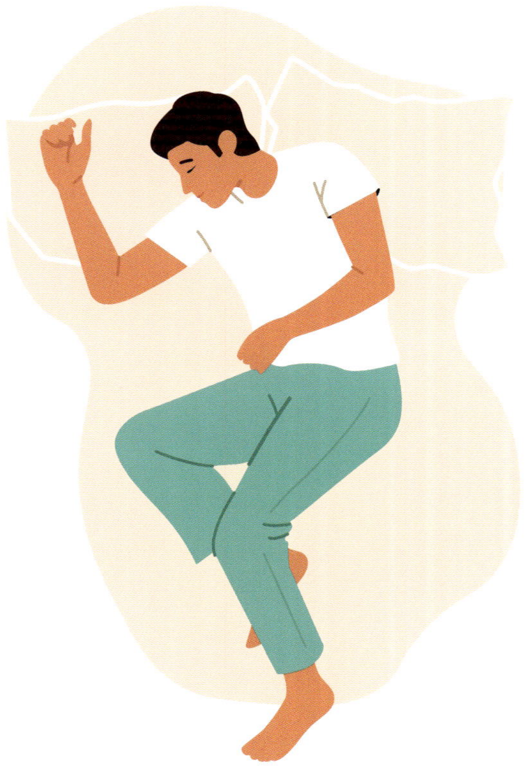

For one in four (24%), the perfect nap should last between 31 minutes and an hour, while one in five (19%) say it should be over an hour.

Britons under the age of 60 (21–29%) are significantly more likely than those over 60 (9%) to say an ideal nap should last more than an hour.

One in five Britons (24%) would like to eliminate the need for sleep if that were possible, while the majority (61%) would not.

Men (31%) are more likely than women (18%) to say they would eliminate the need for sleep, if it were possible, as are younger Britons (35% of 16- to 24-year-olds) compared to their elders (14% of 60+).

29 June 2022

The above information is reprinted with kind permission from YouGov.
YouGov PLC, 2025 © All rights reserved

www.yougov.co.uk

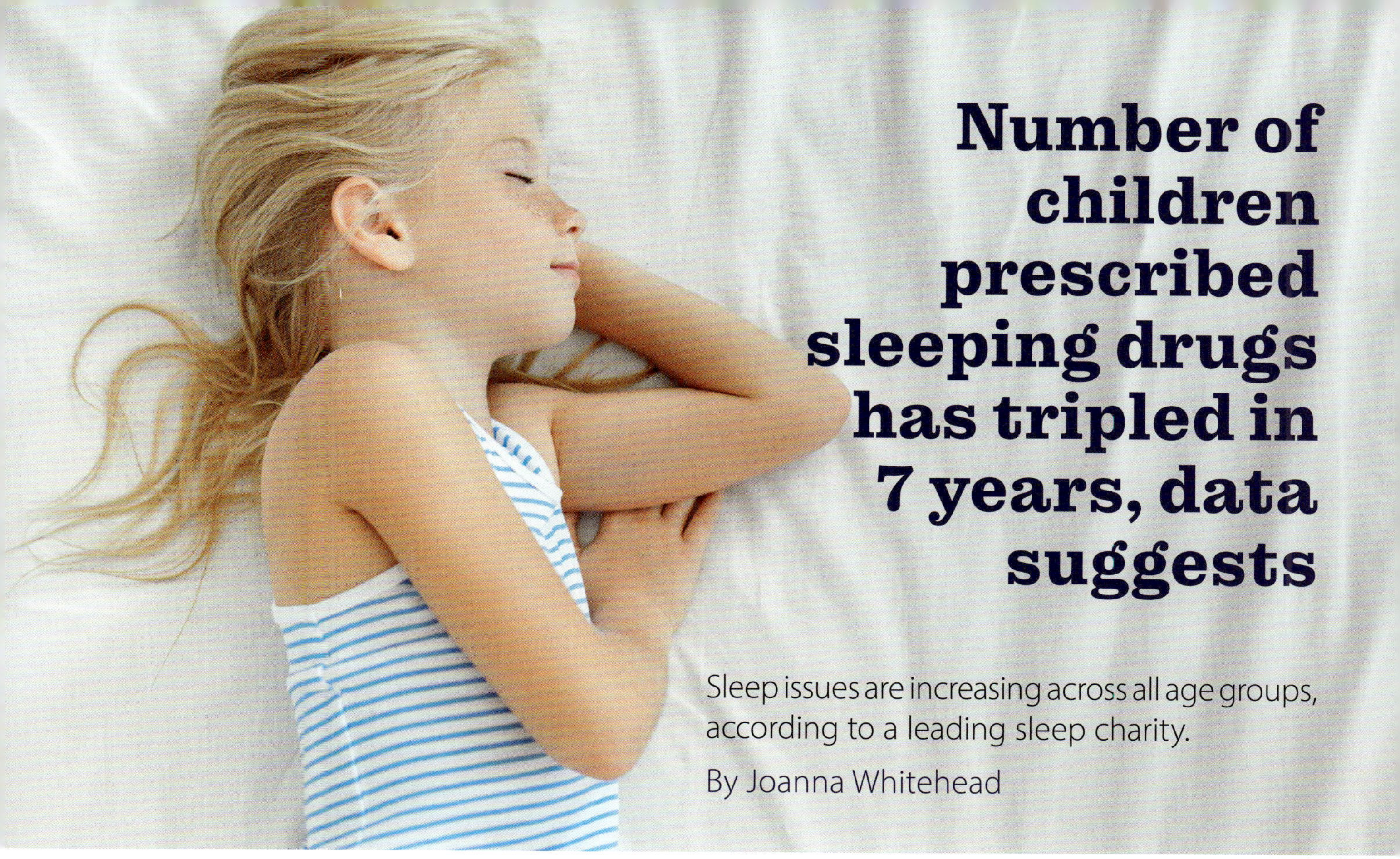

Number of children prescribed sleeping drugs has tripled in 7 years, data suggests

Sleep issues are increasing across all age groups, according to a leading sleep charity.

By Joanna Whitehead

The number of children being prescribed drugs for sleep has almost tripled in the past seven years, prompting concern that medication is being overused due to a lack of support for families.

Synthetic melatonin – a prescription-only drug in the UK – has seen a spike in demand in recent years to help with sleep problems.

Now, an analysis of NHS data obtained under the Freedom of Information Act by *The Pharmaceutical Journal* reveals that 56,002 patients aged 17 or under were prescribed the drug in April 2022 alone.

This compares to just 20,881 in April 2015, an increase of 168%.

National Institute for Health and Care Excellence (NICE) guidelines recommend melatonin for the short-term treatment (up to 13 weeks) of insomnia and jet lag in adults aged 55 years or older.

For children, the treatment is restricted to just one to two weeks in the first instance for those with sleep problems, but only under specialist supervision.

Experts have expressed concern about the sharp increase in children being prescribed the drug.

Vicki Beevers, chief executive and founder of The Sleep Charity, based in Doncaster, Yorkshire, described the rising number of patients on melatonin as 'disappointing'.

'The first line of intervention should always be behavioural… but, unfortunately, many families can't access this; it's an absolute postcode lottery,' she said.

Beevers added that sleep issues were increasing among all age groups, with the pandemic having an impact.

'People were having more screen time, reduced exercise opportunities, a loss of routine and there was increased anxiety,' she said.

Concern about the lack of studies on the long-term effects of taking melatonin and its efficacy in treating sleep problems also remain.

'The concern is that melatonin is not recommended to treat chronic insomnia primarily due to lack of data on its safety and efficacy,' Dr Neomi A Shah, a professor in the department of medicine, division of pulmonary, critical care and sleep medicine at the Icahn School of Medicine at Mount Sinai, told *The Independent*. 'Yet, it is being used by the general public to treat insomnia with limited to no success.'

According to the NHS, reported side effects of melatonin include headaches, dizziness, nausea, irritability and sleepiness, while the Mayo Clinic adds that less common side effects can include 'short-term feelings of depression, confusion or disorientation, mood swings, increased risk of seizures, diarrhoea and an increased chance of urinary incontinence at night'.

Steve Tomlin, director of the Children's Medicines Centre and associate chief pharmacist at Great Ormond Street Hospital, told *The Pharmaceutical Journal* that it was 'far too easy' for children to continue on with using melatonin once it has been tried, because it has had 'some effect'.

'That doesn't mean it is needed long term,' he said.

28 November 2022

The above information is reprinted with kind permission from *The Independent*.
© independent.co.uk 2025

www.independent.co.uk

It's almost impossible to keep teens off their phones in bed – but new research shows it really does affect their sleep

An article from The Conversation.

By Rachael Taylor, Professor, Department of Medicine, University of Otago

Parents of children and teenagers have long been warned about the dangers of screen time and digital devices before bed – the worry being that screens could harm the sleep patterns of young people.

But do screens really hurt the length and quality of sleep?

Our new research found that using screens in bed was worse for sleep than using screens for hours before going to bed.

Sleep guidelines recommend no screen use in the hour or two before bed. But we found screen time in the two hours before bed had little impact on young people's sleep. Instead, it was screen time once in bed that caused problems.

Using cameras to track device usage and sleep, we found using a device in bed could cause more harm than screen time right up to bedtime.

These findings challenge long-held assumptions about screen time at night and could help parents improve the quality of their children's sleep.

Connecting sleep and screens

A number of global organisations recommend adolescents stop using devices in the hour or two before bed, and instead undertake activities like reading a book or quiet time with the family.

But these recommendations are based on research with a number of limitations. The studies were designed in such a way that researchers could link sleep and screens. But they don't tell us if changes in how young people used screens had an affect on the length or quality of sleep.

Most of the existing research also used questionnaires to assess both screen time and sleep. Questionnaires are unlikely to capture true screen time accurately, particularly if you are interested in knowing more than just how long an adolescent has spent on their device.

To address some of these weaknesses in the previous research, we asked 85 adolescents aged between 11 and 14 to wear a body camera on their chest for the three hours before bed, for four nights.

These cameras faced outwards and accurately captured when, what and how adolescents used their screens. Because we were interested in overnight screen time as well, a second infrared camera was placed on a tripod in the teenagers bedroom and captured their screen time while in bed. The research participants also wore an actigraph – a watch-sized device that objectively measured screen time.

Teen nighttime activity

It quickly became obvious the adolescents spent a lot of their screen time while in bed.

Our analysis looked at two time periods – from the two hours before they got into bed, and from once they were in bed (clearly under the covers) until they put their devices down and were clearly trying to go to sleep.

Our data showed 99% of the adolescents used screens in the two hours before bed, more than half once they were in bed, and a third even after first trying to go to sleep for the night. Just one teenager did not use screens before bed on any of the four nights.

The screen time before they got into bed had little impact on their sleep that night. However, screen time once in bed did impair their sleep. It stopped them from going to sleep for about half an hour, and reduced the amount of sleep they got that night.

This was particularly true for more interactive screen activities like gaming and multitasking – when they use more than one device at the same time (like watching a movie on Netflix on a laptop while playing Xbox on a gaming device).

In fact, every additional ten minutes of this type of screen time reduced the amount of sleep they got that night by almost the same amount – nine minutes.

Revisiting guidelines

Our research was an observational study looking at the established screen habits of young people.

The next step to better understanding this will be to conduct experiments that can actually prove different types and timings of screen time affect sleep.

That said, what we have already found challenges existing guidelines. Screens at night may not be the bogey man they have been made out to be. But allowing young people to have screens in bed can be detrimental to their quality of sleep.

So the simple message might be to keep those devices out of the bedroom.

3 September 2024

THE CONVERSATION

The above information is reprinted with kind permission from The Conversation.
© 2010-2025, The Conversation Trust (UK) Limited

www.theconversation.com

Looking at phone screen before bed is not as harmful to sleep as believed, study says

Blue light from phones, TVs, tablets and computers has long been said to negatively impact our sleep.

By Nicole Vassell

Late-night TikTok watchers can breathe a sigh of relief, as a new study has claimed that the light emitted from smartphones does not have a significant effect on sleep quality.

It has long been advised that those hoping to get a quality night of sleep should avoid using devices such as phones and tablets, and watching TV before bed because of the blue light they produce.

Blue light has been said to suppress melatonin, which is the light-reactive hormone that assists sleep and a human's circadian rhythm, or internal 24-hour clock.

However, a new report published in the medical journal *Sleep Medicine Reviews* has questioned this conclusion, stating that the effect of screens on the ability to fall asleep is not as great as we think.

'If we stand back and look at all of the factors that can be harmful to our sleep, screens are overrated,' said Michael Gradisar, a clinical psychologist who co-wrote the paper.

'There's no evidence from 11 studies conducted across the world that screen light in the hour before bed makes it harder to fall asleep.'

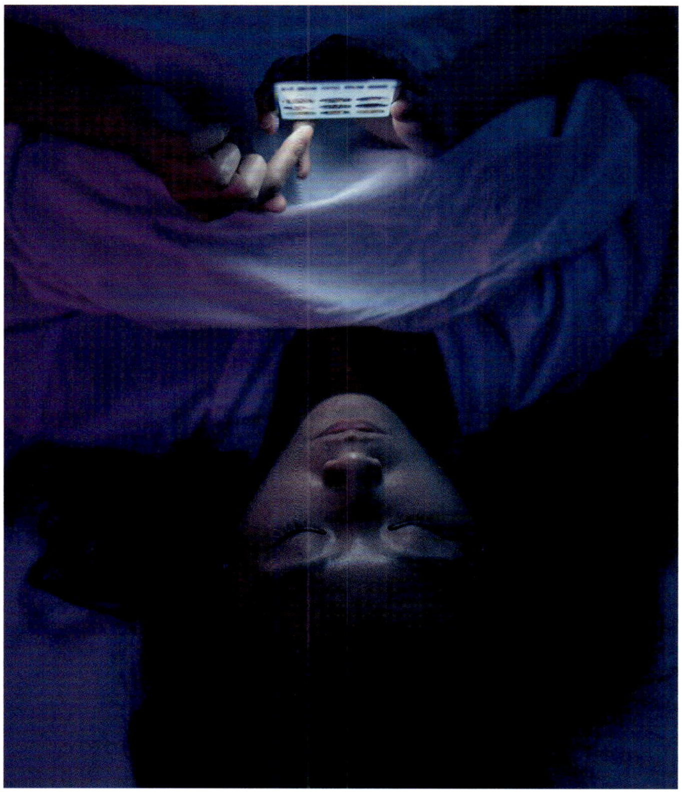

As reported in *The Times*, the biggest effect was seen in one study carried out a decade ago, which found that screens delayed people getting to sleep by only 10 minutes.

'One has to ask, does 10 minutes really make a difference?' Gradisar said.

According to Gradisar and the researchers, the most crucial factor that affects a person's sleep is the time they finally nod off. This may suggest that it is a person's distraction by the device, delaying their slumber, rather than the device itself that impacts sleep.

Still, many researchers note that screen light may affect people differently, with some reacting more strongly to its effects.

Russell Foster, professor of circadian neuroscience at Oxford who isn't connected with the study, has also downplayed the impact of blue light on sleep, adding: 'There's no evidence that the blue lights from screens have any significant impact at all.'

Earlier this year, a study by the University of Basel recorded similar findings and suggested that screen blue light does not greatly affect a person's sleep-wake cycle.

Dr Christine Blume, a psychologist at the Swiss university's Centre for Chronobiology, explained to *Medical News Today* that blue light itself is not massively important on a person's sleep rhythm, but recommended that people reduce their exposure to short-wavelength light in general, regardless of its colour.

'Our results support the findings of many other studies that the light-sensitive ganglion cells are most important for the human internal clock,' Blume said.

'Therefore, short-wavelength light – misleadingly often termed 'blue light' – should be reduced in the evening, for example by dimming computer screens and using a night-shift mode.

'Avoiding screen time before bed can also help, as the things we do on our phones often delay sleep.'

5 June 2024

The above information is reprinted with kind permission from *The Independent*.

© independent.co.uk 2025

www.independent.co.uk

Chapter 3

Building Healthy Sleep Habits

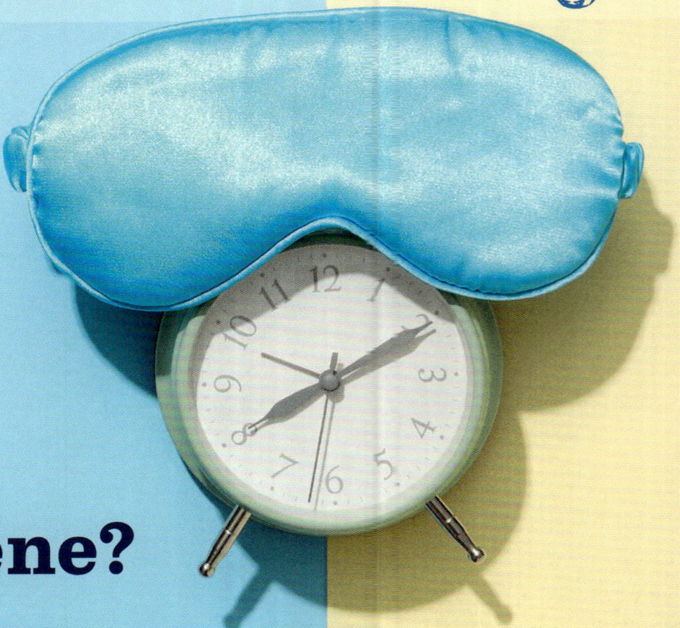

What is sleep hygiene?

By Dr. Sandip Banerjee

Sleep hygiene refers to a set of behavioural and environmental practices aimed at promoting high-quality sleep and maintaining overall health. Quality sleep is essential for cognitive function, emotional stability, physical wellbeing, and disease prevention. Poor sleep hygiene can result in sleep disturbances, reduced productivity, and various health complications. Understanding and implementing proper sleep hygiene practices can significantly enhance sleep quality and wellbeing. This blog will explore sleep hygiene, explaining its role in promoting better sleep, its impact on health, and how to improve sleep quality through simple lifestyle changes.

Importance of sleep hygiene

Sleep is a biological necessity that affects nearly every aspect of health. Proper sleep hygiene ensures the body follows a consistent sleep-wake cycle, optimising physical and mental restoration. On the other hand, poor sleep hygiene can contribute to chronic sleep deprivation, leading to serious health issues such as cardiovascular diseases, metabolic disorders, weakened immunity, and impaired cognitive function. Establishing a structured sleep routine and having a conducive sleep environment can improve short-term and long-term health outcomes.

Mechanism behind sleep

The human body operates on a circadian rhythm, an internal clock that regulates sleep-wake cycles over 24 hours. Exposure to light influences the secretion of melatonin, a hormone responsible for inducing sleep. Disruptions to this natural cycle, such as inconsistent sleep schedules or excessive screen time before bed, can lead to sleep disturbances.

Additionally, sleep occurs in cycles consisting of different stages: light sleep, deep sleep, and rapid eye movement (REM) sleep. Each stage plays a vital role in physical and cognitive restoration. Insufficient or fragmented sleep can impair memory consolidation, emotional regulation, and immune function.

Factors affecting sleep hygiene

Several factors influence sleep hygiene, ranging from lifestyle habits to environmental conditions. These factors can enhance or disrupt sleep quality, making it essential to understand and regulate them effectively.

Consistency in sleep schedule

Maintaining a regular sleep schedule helps to regulate the body's circadian rhythm, which governs the sleep-wake cycle. Going to bed and waking up at the same time daily strengthens the internal clock, making it easier to fall and stay asleep. Irregular sleep schedules disrupt circadian rhythms and contribute to sleep disorders such as insomnia and delayed sleep phase syndrome.

Optimal sleep environment

The sleep environment plays a crucial role in determining sleep quality. Essential components include:

- **Temperature:** A cool room temperature (16–19°C or 60–67°F) facilitates restful sleep.
- **Lighting:** Exposure to bright lights before bedtime can suppress melatonin production. Dimming lights and using blackout curtains create a sleep-conducive environment.
- **Noise reduction:** White noise, earplugs, or soundproofing measures minimise disruptions
- **Bedding quality:** A supportive mattress and comfortable pillows improve sleep quality and prevent discomfort.

Limiting exposure to electronic devices

Electronic screens emit blue light, suppressing melatonin, a hormone essential for sleep. Avoiding screens at least 30–60 minutes before bedtime can prevent delays in sleep onset. Blue light-blocking glasses or night mode settings on devices can mitigate the effects.

Dietary and fluid intake regulation

Certain dietary choices affect sleep quality. Caffeine and nicotine act as stimulants, delaying sleep onset, and should be avoided several hours before bedtime. Heavy meals, especially large, spicy, or fatty meals, can cause discomfort and indigestion that disrupt sleep. Hydration balance is also crucial excessive fluid intake before bed may lead to frequent awakenings due to nighttime urination. Managing these factors promotes better sleep quality.

Pre-sleep relaxation techniques

Practising relaxing activities before bed helps the body prepare for sleep. Reading a low-stimulus book promotes relaxation. Meditation and deep breathing reduce stress and lower cortisol levels. A warm bath or shower helps to lower body temperature, making it easier to fall asleep.

Physical activity and sleep

Regular physical activity enhances sleep quality by reducing stress and promoting deeper sleep stages. However, exercising too close to bedtime may increase alertness and delay sleep onset. Moderate-intensity workouts earlier in the day contribute positively to sleep hygiene.

Managing stress and mental health

Psychological stress such as depression and anxiety, are common barriers to sleep. Adopting coping mechanisms such as journalling, cognitive behavioural therapy (CBT), and guided relaxation can alleviate stress-related sleep disturbances. Establishing a bedtime routine that minimises overthinking can prevent sleep-onset insomnia.

Consequences of poor sleep hygiene

Poor sleep hygiene can lead to various short-term and long-term consequences, impacting physical, mental, and emotional wellbeing.

Cognitive impairment: Lack of quality sleep affects concentration, memory, and decision-making abilities. This results in decreased workplace efficiency, academic struggles, and increased risk of accidents.

Risk of chronic diseases: Persistent poor sleep is associated with various chronic conditions. Sleep deprivation elevates blood pressure and increases the risk of heart disease and stroke. Poor sleep affects insulin sensitivity and glucose metabolism, increasing the likelihood of type 2 diabetes. Disrupted sleep patterns alter hunger hormones, increasing appetite and weight gain.

Mental health disorders: Sleep deprivation is closely linked to mental health conditions such as depression, anxiety, and mood disorders. Chronic sleep issues exacerbate emotional instability and increase susceptibility to psychological distress.

Weakened immune system: Poor sleep hygiene weakens immune function, making the body more susceptible to infections and illnesses. Proper rest is essential for immune system regulation and recovery processes.

Sleep hygiene across different life stages

Sleep hygiene needs vary across different age groups. Implementing age-appropriate strategies enhances overall wellbeing and ensures optimal sleep quality.

Infants and children

Establishing bedtime routines early in life helps to regulate sleep patterns. Consistency in sleep schedules, avoiding overstimulation before bedtime, and a safe sleep environment are crucial for children's sleep hygiene. Parents should ensure that screen exposure is minimised before bedtime and that children associate bedtime with calming activities.

Teenagers

Adolescents experience shifts in their circadian rhythm, leading to later sleep onset and difficulty waking up early. Encouraging good sleep hygiene, such as limiting screen time and maintaining consistent sleep schedules, is essential. Schools and parents should promote awareness about the importance of sufficient sleep for academic performance and mental health.

Adults and elderly individuals

Both adults and elderly individuals face sleep challenges due to lifestyle factors and ageing. Maintaining a consistent sleep schedule, managing stress, and creating a comfortable sleep environment improve sleep quality. Adults should set structured routines and limit work in bed, while elderly individuals benefit from regular physical activity and addressing health conditions like sleep apnoea or restless leg syndrome.

Common misconceptions about sleep hygiene

Sleeping more on weekends to compensate for sleep debt disrupts circadian rhythms, so maintaining a consistent sleep schedule is key for long-term health. While alcohol may make you drowsy, it actually leads to disrupted, poor-quality sleep. Similarly, high-intensity exercise close to bedtime can delay sleep onset by raising heart rate and body temperature, making moderate exercise earlier in the day a better choice for improved sleep.

Practising good sleep hygiene is important for maintaining overall health and wellbeing. Establishing a consistent sleep schedule, optimising the sleep environment, regulating diet and physical activity, and managing stress can improve sleep quality and long-term health outcomes. Understanding the consequences of poor sleep hygiene and implementing necessary lifestyle adjustments can significantly enhance cognitive and physical performance. Prioritising sleep as a core component of health ensures sustainable wellbeing and improved quality of life.

29 January 2025

The above information is reprinted with kind permission from Dr Sandip Banerjee.

© 2025 Dr Sandip Banerjee

www.drsandipbanerjee.co.uk

Tips to improve your sleep

If you experience sleep problems, there are some ideas you can try.

Remember that different things work at different times. So only try what you feel comfortable with, and don't put too much pressure on yourself.

Try to establish a routine

It could help to establish a regular sleeping routine and good sleeping habits. You might need to try different things to find what works for you.

You could try going to bed and waking up at around the same time every day. Or it might help to go to bed only once you feel ready to sleep, but still get up around the same time.

It may also help to do something relaxing just before you go to bed. For example, you could listen to relaxing music.

You might hear some people use the term 'sleep hygiene'. This may include some doctors. This term means having a good routine around your sleep.

'I only go to bed when I feel like I will fall asleep within about 15 minutes or so, no matter what time of night that is, and then I try to get up at the same time every day.'

Don't force yourself to sleep

If you're struggling to get to sleep, try not to force yourself.

Instead, try doing something relaxing in bed. Or get up and do something calming, until you feel tired.

Find ways to relax

If you experience lots of stress, this could affect how well you sleep. Finding ways to relax could help with this. For example, breathing exercises and meditation.

'A nicely made bed helps. If I'm having an awful day, and the only thing I've managed to find the energy to do is make my bed, then that's OK.'

Fill in a sleep diary

You may find it difficult to work out what's affecting your sleep. A sleep diary involves recording information about your sleep habits. This can help you understand your sleep problem and what's affecting it.

If you want to, you can show your sleep diary to healthcare professionals. It could help explain what problems you're having. For example, you could take it with you to a doctor's appointment.

A sleep diary could include information about:

- What time you went to bed and what time you got up
- How long you slept for
- How well you slept, which you could rank on a scale or use pictures or words to describe

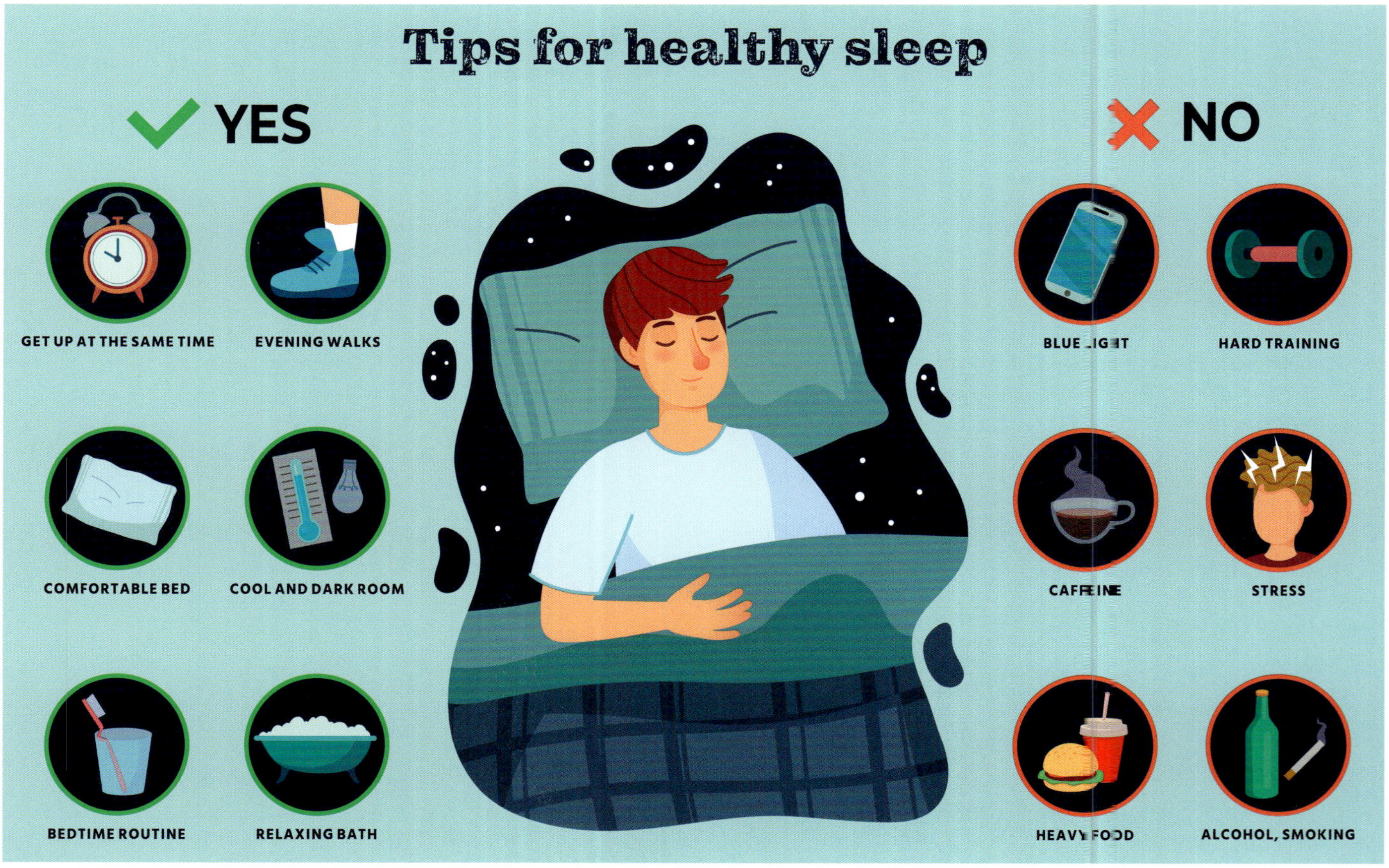

- How many times you woke up in the night, how long you were awake and what you did while you were awake
- Whether you had nightmares, night terrors or sleep paralysis, or sleepwalked during the night
- Whether you slept during the day and for how long
- Any medication you're taking, including the dose and what time you take it
- The amount of caffeine, alcohol or nicotine you have, and at what time of day
- The amount of physical activity you do, and at what time of day
- Your general feelings and moods, including any anxious or repetitive thoughts

You should keep your sleep diary for at least two weeks. It's ok if you don't know the answers to everything. You can make a guess, or leave sections blank.

'I write what's happened, what did or didn't help, anything I need to or scribble to let out anger when the words and the tears are stuck.'

Make your sleeping area more comfortable

You might not have much control over where you sleep. For example, if you're staying in hospital or temporary accommodation. But there might still be small changes you can make, or ask someone to help you with.

These are some ideas you could try:

- Try different temperature, light and noise levels to see what works for you. For example, you could try keeping a light on or using earplugs.
- If silence makes it harder to sleep, listen to music, nature sounds, a podcast or the radio.
- You might find it helpful to try different bedding. For example, a warmer or cooler duvet, or a different pillow.

'Sometimes when I'm trying to fall asleep I don't like being alone with my thoughts. I have found podcasts an amazing comfort – it just keeps my mind occupied enough not to start spiralling, and to fall asleep.'

Think about screens and device settings

Using screens in the evening, including on tablets and mobile phones, can negatively affect your sleep.

It can help to think about when and how you use screens. For example, you could try to:

- Avoid or cut down on using screens shortly before sleep
- Reduce the brightness of any screen you use
- Avoid stimulating activities before going to sleep, such as playing games on a screen
- Reduce distractions by switching on silent, airplane or do not disturb mode, if you can

'Reminding myself that a bad night of sleep won't make or break me (because I can make it through, even if it sucks) has helped a lot to allay stress and anxiety about sleep.'

Look after yourself

Looking after your physical health can help improve your sleep. These are some tips that might help.

Think about your diet

Some types of foods can affect your sleep, including caffeine and sugar. It can also help to avoid eating large meals right before going to bed. Our pages on food and mental health have more information.

Try to do some physical activity

Physical activity can help you sleep, including gentle physical activity. But try not to do this too close to when you want to sleep. Some people find this makes them feel more awake.

Treatment to help with sleep problems

If you're struggling with your sleep, you could speak to your GP for help. They may be able to offer treatments for things that can affect your sleep, including mental health problems.

They'll probably recommend ways to improve your sleep quality without treatment. But if those don't work, then they might suggest these treatments.

Talking therapies

Cognitive behavioural therapy for insomnia (CBT-I) is a type of therapy designed to help with insomnia. If you access CBT-I through the NHS, it is most likely to happen online. But in some areas of the UK it might be available in person.

You may also be offered talking therapy to help with mental health problems that are affecting your sleep. See our pages on talking therapy and counselling for more information.

Medication

In some cases, your GP might offer sleeping pills for a short period. But this is usually only if you have severe problems with insomnia.

There are also medications that can help with other sleep disorders, such as narcolepsy or sleep apnoea. You can speak to your GP about this.

Referral to a sleep clinic

Sleep clinics can assess sleep problems. This could be by using equipment at home or staying overnight for an assessment. To access a sleep clinic, you'll usually need a referral from your GP.

December 2024

The above information is reprinted with kind permission from Mind.
© 2025 Mind
www.mind.org.uk

Sleepy girl mocktail and mouth tape? Experts debunk top 4 TikTok 'sleep hacks'

Over 49K TikTok videos share 'sleep hacks, ' but how accurate are they?

Each month, there are, on average, 9.9K Google searches for 'why can't I fall asleep?' But why do some of us struggle? There are a few different factors that can contribute to poor sleep quality, including bad sleep habits, stress and anxiety, health conditions or even the food and drink you consume.

Recently, there has been an influx of TikTok videos sharing some familiar and some peculiar ways to fall asleep. In fact, there has been a whopping 49K videos using the hashtag #sleephacks.

Unfortunately, most of the videos cannot be accredited to qualified health professionals, which raises concerns on how beneficial some of these 'hacks' can be. Because of this, bed specialists from Happy Beds have teamed up with medical expert Dr Deborah Lee at Dr Fox Online Pharmacy to crack the code on some of the most popular sleep remedies on TikTok.

Top 4 TikTok 'Sleep Hacks'

1. Be cautious with mouth taping

Rex Isap, bed specialist at Happy Beds explains, 'Mouth tape has taken the internet by storm, and with over 63K TikTok videos and 2.9K Google searches per month, it is definitely something the UK is exploring when it comes to improving their sleep, but it is concerning that not every user is researching into the possible negatives of using the technique'.

Dr Deborah Lee has shared her thoughts on whether it is beneficial and some warnings to users.

'Many health claims are made about nocturnal mouth taping. It is said to help you sleep better, lower your blood pressure and boost your immunity. Some advocate it to help reduce snoring and as a treatment for obstructive sleep apnoea (OSA).

'But mouth taping also has its drawbacks. These include skin irritation around the mouth, pain removing the tape, anxiety and sleep disruption. In anyone with acid reflux, if your mouth is taped shut it might increase the risk of aspirating stomach acids. Some people have reduced airflow through the nose due to enlarged tonsils or adenoids, a deviated nasal septum, nasal polyps or inflammation due to allergies. Blocking the mouth can mean they struggle to get enough air in through their nose, which is dangerous for your health.'

2. Be precise with a sleepy girl mocktail

If you find yourself lying awake at night, some TikTok videos suggest trying the 'sleepy girl mocktail', crowned as a sure-fire way to drift off into a deep sleep with over 11K TikTok videos to date.

The sleep-inducing drink contains cherry juice, one tablespoon of magnesium powder and sparkling water. Dr Deborah Lee has analysed the ingredients to decipher if there is any real benefit:

'There may be some benefits to trying this drink before bedtime but there is no robust medical evidence to show it is effective.'

Dr Deborah explains why one of the key ingredients could make you feel sleepy: 'Tart cherries – real name Montmorency cherries – have been shown in one small (20 patients) randomised double-blind placebo-controlled study to significantly raise the blood level of the sleep hormone, melatonin. It also improved total sleep time and sleep efficiency (the time spent in bed asleep). Tart cherries are a specific type of cherry, known to have a high concentration of the sleep hormone, melatonin, so there is a plausible biochemical reason why it might work.'

'Magnesium may help sleep as it supports mental and physical relaxation, and it is a muscle relaxant. However, the NHS recommends men and women take no more than 420mg and 300mg of magnesium per day respectively. One tablespoon of magnesium glycinate as in the 'Sleepy Girl Mocktail' contains 500mg of magnesium. Sparkling water,

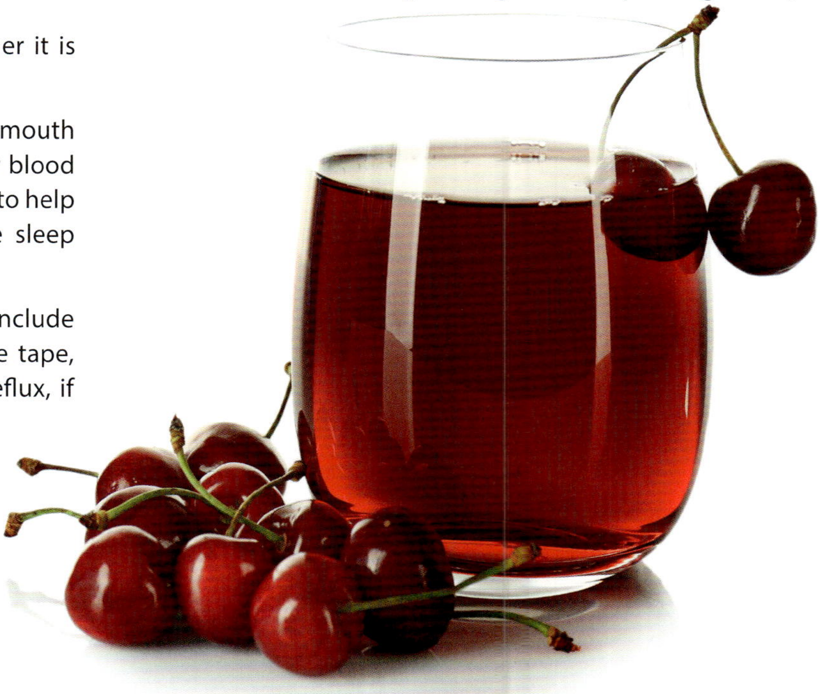

also part of the mocktai , is a source of magnesium in itself. Take note that you can ncrease your magnesium levels by eating foods such as whole grains, spinach, quinoa, dark chocolate, edamame beans and avocado.'

3. Struggling to sleep? Try 4-7-8 breathwork

Rex says, 'Breathing techniques aren't revolutionary in the world of relaxation, but there is one strategy that has swept across the internet with its claims to make you fall asleep in under two minutes.'

Allegedly used in the armed forces to fall asleep in noisy locations the 4-7-8 breathwork trend totted up a whopping 45K videos on TikTok. Rex explains how it works: 'The technique includes laying on your back, relaxing your facial muscles and then following these three simple steps; inhaling for 4 seconds, holding your breath for 7 seconds and then exhaling for 8 seconds. This is then repeated until you fall asleep.'

Dr Deborah explains that this type of breathwork is designed to relieve stress and help you to relax.

'This is a specific type of breathing called diaphragmatic breathing. Research exists to show that controlled breathing can lower stress and stress is a major cause of insomnia.'

'Doing diaphragmatic breathing means breathing in by sucking in your rib cage. When you do this, you are expanding your chest to take in air by raising the diaphragm, the sheet of muscle that divides your chest from your abdomen, activating the vagus nerve, which is the main parasympathetic nerve in the body. The parasympathetic nervous system (PSNS) is one of the body's anti-anxiety pathways. When stimulated, it slows the heart and breathing rate and makes us feel less stressed and more relaxed. The important thing is to breathe in, hold it, and then breathe out for longer than you breathed in. This is vital otherwise you will be over breathing and resting carbon dioxide which makes things worse not better!'

4. The alphabet method comes in handy

Another popular trend includes playing the alphabet game in your head to encourage you to drift off, making it one of the simplest strategies floating around the internet.

It includes thinking of something for each letter of the alphabet; this could be something you are grateful for, names of celebrities, or fruits, etc. The idea is to give your brain a distraction, enough to fall asleep but not too much to be over-stimulating.

Dr Deborah explains why this method is expert-approved to help you drift off into a peaceful sleep:

'The amygdala is found in the temporal lobe of the brain. This has a major role in processing emotions. At night, this may become overactive, which is made worse by poor sleep quality and sleep deprivation. Concentrating on a topic, such as the alphabet game, is a good way of focussing your thoughts.

'Any activity where we take control of our thoughts and do not allow the amygdala to take over is likely to help us sleep.

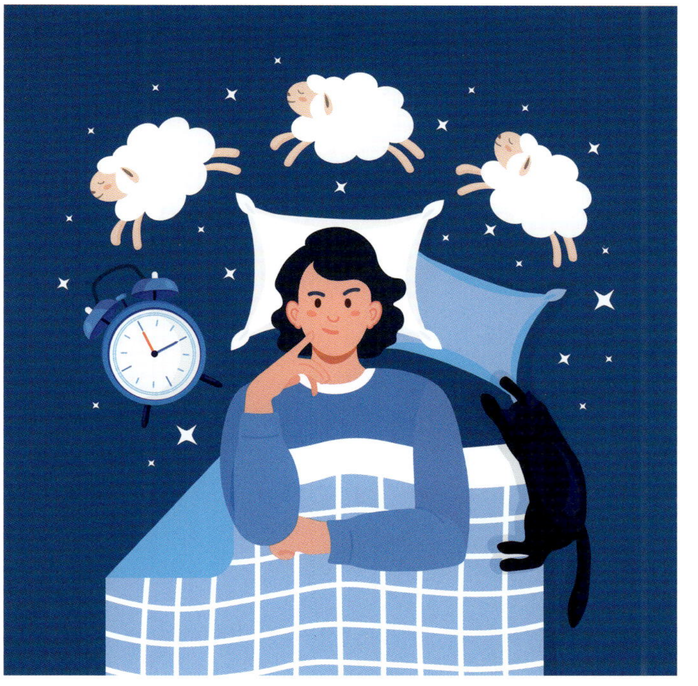

When it comes to sleep, you must learn to control your thoughts and not let your thoughts control you.'

Josie Potts, Head of Merchandise and sleep expert at Happy Beds has listed some of the key things you can do each day to help you sleep:

- Set a bedtime routine: Go to bed and wake up at the same time every day (even at weekends).
- Make sure your bed is comfortable: Ensure your bed is comfortable, supportive and has plenty of room, and that your mattress is right for you.
- Create a relaxing environment: Your room should be dark, quiet and free from distractions. No TV, phones or electrical devices. Your bedroom should be associated with sleep.
- Avoid tech before bed: Avoid using your phone or social media just before bed. Blue lights from electronics can cause your brain to become more alert, meaning you struggle to fall asleep.
- Try relaxation techniques: Having a bath, spending a little time on a skincare routine, or even meditating before bed can help. Creating a routine signal to your brain that sleep is coming, making it easier for you to switch off.
- Exercise: Being active throughout the day helps your body get into a consistent routine and also helps ensure you're tired at the right time of night.
- Avoid food and drink triggers: Avoid caffeine, sugary foods, and big meals before bedtime. Alcohol should also be avoided. Although it initially makes you sleepy, it can disrupt sleep.

10 April 2025

The above information is reprinted with kind permission from *London Daily News*.
© 2025 London Daily News Ltd
www.londondaily.news

How to sleep better

This content mentions depression and anxiety, which some people may find triggering.

HEAL: The four pillars of good sleep

There are four main things that affect the quality of our sleep:

- Health
- Environment
- Attitude
- Lifestyle

Good sleep doesn't just mean lots of sleep: it means the right kind of sleep.

Sleep affects our ability to use language, maintain attention, understand what we are reading, and summarise what we are hearing; if we compromise on our sleep, we compromise on our performance, our mood, and our interpersonal relationships. Sleep has also been shown to protect the immune system. The amount that each of us needs is different. However, it's recommended that a healthy adult should sleep, on average, between seven and nine hours a night.

The important thing is that you get good quality sleep. The following advice can help to HEAL your sleep problems.

Health

As anyone who has tried to get to sleep with a blocked nose or headache knows, physical health problems can stop you from getting a good night's sleep.

Speaking to your GP or pharmacist about appropriate medication can help with this. Try to avoid taking medication without speaking to a medical professional, as sometimes the medication itself can stop you from sleeping properly if it's not right for you.

Mental health problems like anxiety and depression can also affect our sleep. In these cases, a combined approach to tackle both the mental health issue and the poor sleep is often the most effective method of treatment. Speak to your GP or mental health worker (if you have one) for advice on this, or have a look at the 'Attitude' and 'Lifestyle' sections of this guide for general ways to maintain good mental wellbeing.

Environment

The bedroom should be somewhere that we associate with sleep.

Where possible, try to remove distractions from your bedroom. It's better to watch TV, play computer games and eat in another room. This will help you to relax with no distractions in your bedroom.

Be aware of the presence of gadgets and electronics, such as computers, phones, tablets and TVs. The 'blue light' displays suppress melatonin production – the hormone that helps you sleep. The suppression of melatonin causes sleep disruption. It's a good idea not to use these devices two hours before you go to sleep to reduce their effect on your sleeping.

Although we are all different and have our own personal preferences, the common factors that can affect our sleep are light, noise and temperature. Too much light or noise can prevent you from falling asleep or staying asleep. If you can't control the amount of light and noise, such as light from a street lamp or noise from a neighbour's music, you could try using an eye mask or ear plugs.

The temperature of the room is also important. A heater or thicker duvet can help if you regularly find yourself too cold at night, or a thinner cover or opening a window can help if you're too hot. If you are struggling to work out the best sleep environment for you, then it can be useful to keep a sleep diary (there's one at the end of this guide) to keep track of the conditions that helped you get a good night's sleep.

Attitude

Lying awake in bed, particularly before an important day, can make us worry. However, this worry then makes it harder for us to get to sleep.

Relaxation techniques can help you to unwind at these times. Alternatively, instead of staying in bed and getting more and more frustrated, you could get up and make yourself a warm drink (avoid coffee, tea or any other caffeine drinks) and return to bed when you feel sleepier.

If you keep having problems sleeping for more than a month, you could speak with your GP about the possibility of using Cognitive Behavioural Therapy (CBT). CBT is used to treat some mental health problems. It can encourage a more positive attitude, which can then help to break the cycle of negative thoughts causing your lack of sleep, and thus can help you to develop a healthier sleep pattern. In England you can self-refer for NHS talking therapies service (which may help reduce unnecessary use of GP time and speed referrals if talking treatments are appropriate).

Alternatively, practices like mindfulness (a type of meditation) can help by reducing stress and anxiety levels. Mindfulness can be practised without a GP prescription.

Lifestyle

There are many things that you can do every day to improve the quality of your sleep.

Eating rice, oats and dairy products can produce chemicals that increase our desire to sleep. However, food and drink containing lots of caffeine or sugar can keep you awake, so drinking less tea and coffee and eating less chocolate and other sugary foods late in the day might help you to sleep better.

Although it can make you feel tired and can help you get to sleep, alcohol impairs the quality of your sleep and makes you more likely to wake up during the night as the effects wear off, and you may need to go to the toilet frequently or get up to drink water if you are dehydrated.

Exercising on a regular basis is thought to help us sleep, as, among other things, it can help to reduce anxiety and relieve

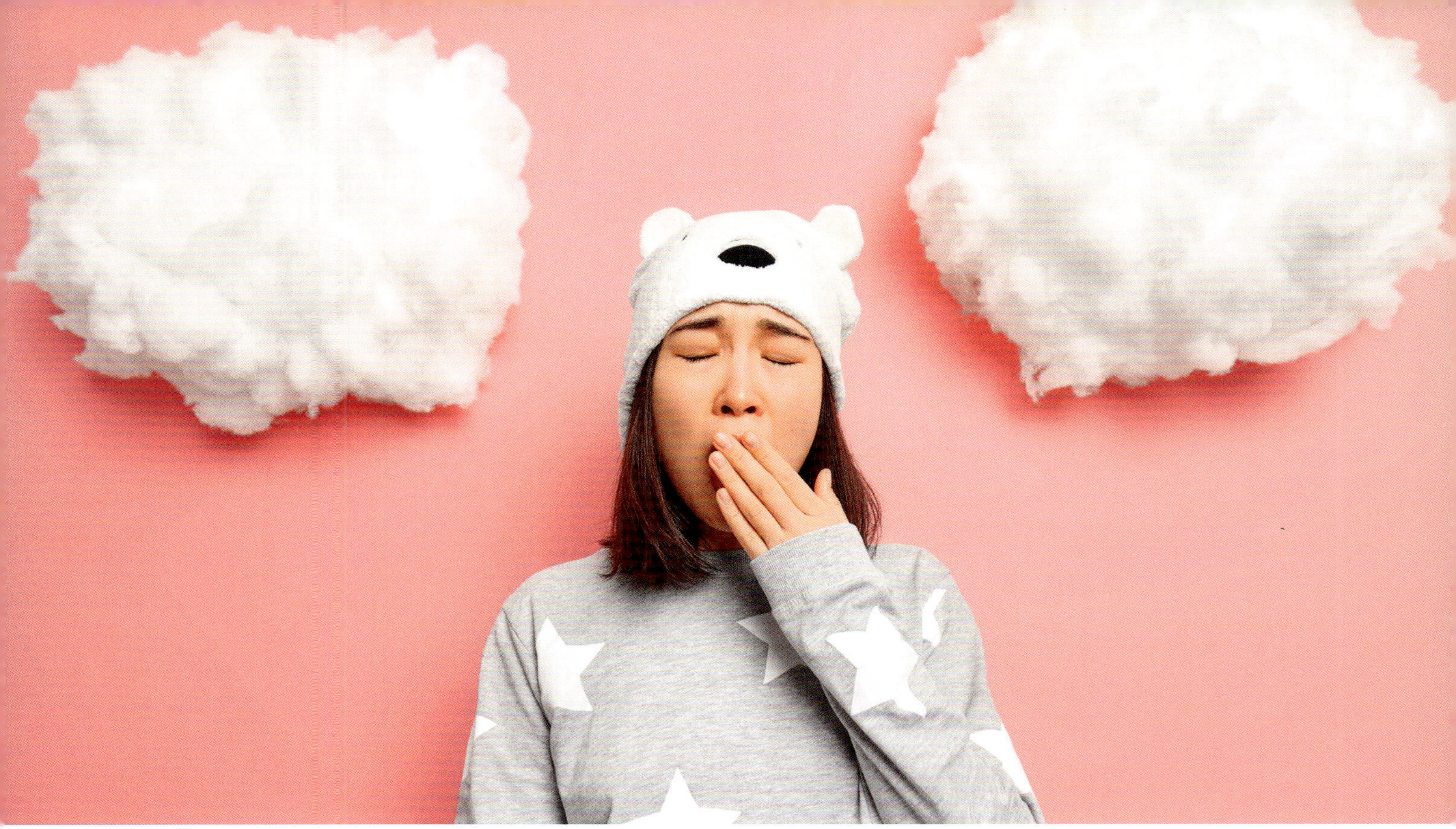

stress. It is, however, important to exercise at the right time. Exercising earlier in the day is better, as exercise increases the body's adrenaline production, making it more difficult to sleep if done just before bedtime.

Sleep disorders – the problems they cause and possible solutions

Below are some of the most common sleep problems, with techniques that can be used to treat them.

Insomnia

Insomnia is a condition where you are regularly unable to fall asleep or remain asleep for a long enough period of time. As a result, insomnia can have a negative effect on your mood, energy levels, concentration, relationships, ability to stay awake throughout the day, and ability to complete simple daily tasks.

One of the most widely used and successful therapies is Cognitive Behavioural Therapy (CBT); for an easy introduction, read *Overcoming Insomnia and Sleep Problems* by Colin Espie or ask your local GP or sleep clinic for advice on other CBT books or courses. Regular daytime or early evening exercise can also be a great way to combat insomnia as it helps to reduce anxiety and stress, as can practices such as mindfulness.

Using sleep medication, such as sleeping pills, is common. However, these types of medication are only available by prescription from your GP and you can become reliant on them the longer you use them. Speak to your GP if your insomnia persists.

Sleepwalking

Sleepwalking happens during deep sleep, meaning people can rarely remember doing it. As well as getting out of bed and walking, some people do tasks in their sleep, such as cleaning. Sleepwalking is far more common in children than in adults.

Sleepwalking is not dangerous unless you start doing risky activities in your sleep. It is often related to stress or lack of sleep, or (in adults) drinking alcohol, so it is important to try and get regular, good-quality sleep by looking at the HEAL factors mentioned earlier in this guide.

Night terrors

A night terror is different to a nightmare. It occurs during deep sleep, meaning that you rarely remember it. Often an extreme and frightening experience, night terrors make your heart beat faster and might cause you to sweat or scream. Night terrors often begin in childhood, but rarely continue into adulthood.

Little is known about how to treat people who have regular night terrors, although, in some cases, they can be linked to a traumatic experience. If this is the case, and your night terrors are affecting your everyday life or ability to sleep, your GP might be able to refer you for therapy to help you deal with the underlying trauma.

Snoring

Snoring is a very common problem, affecting 41.5% of adults in the UK. Snoring is a breathing problem, rather than sleep problem, and happens when a blockage in the airway causes the organs that help us breathe to vibrate.

Nasal strips can help by widening the nasal passage and improving the airflow when breathing. It is also better to sleep on your side, as sleeping on your back can cause your tongue to fall backwards and partially block your airflow. Drinking less alcohol, exercising more regularly, and taking steps to lose weight (if you are overweight) can also reduce your snoring.

Sleep apnoea

Sleep apnoea causes shallow breathing or pauses in breathing that may last up to 30 seconds at a time. In most cases, you will begin to breathe normally again, often making a loud snort or choking sound to clear your airway. People with sleep apnoea can wake up frequently throughout the night feeling sweaty with a dry mouth and a headache.

Unlike snoring, it is more important to treat sleep apnoea in order to prevent the brain from being deprived of oxygen. A continuous positive airway pressure (CPAP) device can help by easing your airflow. Your GP will be able to recommend where you can get an assessment for a CPAP device.

Top tips from the sleep doctor

Don't get caught napping!

If you have trouble sleeping, you may feel tempted to catch up on sleep by taking naps. However, unless you're feeling dangerously sleepy (while driving or operating machinery, for instance), this usually does more harm than good as it makes it more difficult to sleep at night. If you feel tired during the day, get up and take a walk around, get some fresh air, or do something challenging for a short while, like a crossword or a Sudoku.

If you're not tired, get up

If you're finding it difficult to get to sleep, don't just lie there worrying. Get up for a few minutes and get a drink (no sugar or caffeine, remember!), and go back to bed when you're feeling a bit sleepier.

Set yourself a 'get fit' plan

Eating healthily and getting regular exercise are great ways of helping yourself sleep better. However, plan your meals and exercise to avoid exercising or eating a big meal after mid-evening: doing either of these too close to your bedtime can stop you from sleeping.

Don't stress it!

Thinking about sleep too much or trying to force yourself to sleep will only keep you awake. Learning how to relax both your body and mind instead will help you to get to sleep much more easily.

Keep a sleep diary

The amount of noise, light, and distractions, what and when you eat, and the temperature of your bedroom can affect how well you sleep. Keeping a sleep diary to make a note of what the conditions were when you went to bed the night before can be useful for letting you look back and see what has and what hasn't worked for you. It also helps you to see how your sleep varies from night to night, and might help you note patterns in your sleeping.

Random sleep facts

- The Beatles' song *Yesterday* came to Paul McCartney in a dream. It was only when no one he spoke to recognised the tune that he realised he had written it himself.
- Driver sleepiness may contribute to around 20% of accidents on long journeys.
- Pythons sleep for up to 18 hours a day. Giraffes generally sleep for less than two.

Further information

Sleepio – An organisation dedicated to helping people sleep better, co-founded by Professor Colin Espie, Director of the University of Oxford Sleep Research Centre and the 'top tips' sleep doctor in this guide. The Sleepio website includes information about various sleep problems.

Your local GP – If you continue to be concerned about the amount and quality of sleep you are having, and the effects it is having on other aspects of your life, you should speak to your GP, who will be able to help and provide further guidance and support.

British Snoring & Sleep Apnoea Association – A not-for-profit organisation dedicated to helping snorers and their bed partners improve their sleep.

Be Mindful – Be Mindful to make courses in mindfulness meditation available to everyone who wants or needs them. This site provides useful information on what mindfulness is and the different mindfulness-based courses available. You can also search for mindfulness courses near you, or sign up for the specially developed online course.

British Sleep Society – A charity for medical, scientific and healthcare workers dealing with sleep disorders in the UK.

Sleep diary

Working out the reasons why you might have problems sleeping can be difficult. Keeping a sleep diary can help you keep track of when you slept well or poorly, and the possible reasons why that happened.

To complete the sleep diary, simply read and answer the following questions for at least a week.

Remember, this diary is your personal record of how well you slept and why, so be honest!

Questions for the sleep diary

1. How did you sleep last night?
2. What time did you go to bed?
3. Approximately how long did it take you to get to sleep?
4. How many times did you wake up during the night?
5. What time did you wake up?
6. How long did you sleep for in total?
7. What did you eat or drink (if anything) within four hours of going to bed (e.g., cup of tea/coffee/milky drink, glass of wine/beer, sleeping pills, dinner), and how long before bed did you have it?
8. What was the temperature outside and in your bedroom?
9. What light sources were there when you went to sleep?
10. How much noise was there when you went to sleep?
11. What activities did you do before you went to sleep?
12. Any other comments?
13. How well did you feel throughout the next day (1 = awful, 5 = average, 10 = great)? Include a description, if appropriate (e.g., drowsy, grumpy, spaced out).

The above information is reprinted with kind permission from The Mental Health Foundation.

© 2025 Mental Health Foundation

www.mentalhealth.org.uk

Sleep tips for exam success

Getting enough sleep is vital to feeling and performing your best, which makes a good night's rest particularly vital around exam time. Our Surrey sleep experts share tips and advice to help you sleep better during your exams.

How to sleep better during exams

Wake up fresh and prepared every morning:

1. Make time for sleep

The most important thing is to remember to schedule time for sleep. When you have to get up at a certain time, count back the number of hours you want to sleep and then add half an hour. This time becomes the scheduled time to switch the lights out. The extra half an hour is important - we often forget about the time it takes to brush teeth, set the alarm clock and so on.

2. Watch what you eat and when

Eating late meals because you have been studying all day will alter your internal clock and impair sleep. Although you should try not to go to bed hungry, try to have a big dinner before 7pm and then a smaller snack in the evening if you are still hungry. It's thought that certain foods help sleep; turkey, milk, bananas, and walnuts all contain tryptophan, which the body uses to make melatonin.

3. Limit caffeinated drinks

Although the impact of caffeine varies from person to person, try avoiding all sources of caffeine from 3pm and adjust if needed. Remember caffeine isn't just in coffee – it's also in things like tea, chocolate, and fizzy drinks.

4. Make your bedroom a place of rest

Checking emails or doing some last-minute revision in bed may stop your brain associating the bedroom as a place of quiet rest and, instead, the bed becomes associated as a place of cognitive arousal. This can make it hard to initiate sleep, so remove all distracting items from the bedroom area.

5. Don't use your smartphone in bed

Electronic devices emit noise and light; both will stop you sleeping. LCD screens on phones and tablets emit light that is blue enriched. This light influences the body's internal clock (circadian rhythm) and delays the release of the 'sleep hormone' melatonin. Without melatonin, although you can sleep, the sleep you achieve will be light and non-refreshing. Light can also make you feel more alert, again training the brain to perceive the bed as a place of cognitive arousal.

6. Have a bedtime routine

Doing exercise is a great way to relax during the exam period, as it causes the release of endorphins and improves your mood. However, the endorphins released from exercise can also impair sleep. As such, try to avoid exercising within two hours of bedtime. Instead, use those few hours to create a relaxing bedtime routine – perhaps by having a bath with lavender oil, or sitting and reading a book.

7. Clear your head before bed

There's some truth in the old saying that taking a problem to bed means you wake up with the solution – but don't let the problem keep you awake.

Sitting and ruminating over thoughts of the day will keep the brain active, so try keeping a notebook by your bed to write thoughts down before sleep instead. Meditation and breathing exercises can also help.

If you can't drop off, don't stay in bed trying to force yourself to sleep. Instead, employ the 15-minute rule: if you can't sleep after what feels like 15 minutes, get up, leave the bedroom, and read or relax somewhere else. Only return to the room when you feel sleepy again.

8. Remember – one night of bad sleep won't hurt

Your day may be more difficult and you might need more coffee to function, but you will make it through the day after one night of poor sleep. Sleep is an autonomic function – you can't force yourself to sleep, so worrying about not sleeping or the effect of not sleeping on the following day will impair sleep.

Try not to nap, but if you need to, keep any naps to less than 30 minutes in length and don't take them after 3pm. Remember, after a night of poor sleep, you are more likely to sleep the following night!

13 March 2024

The above information is reprinted with kind permission from the University of Surrey.
© 2025 University of Surrey

www.surrey.ac.uk

Design a restful revision space

Draw a layout of your ideal revision corner and your ideal bedroom space for sleep.

Label where you would keep books and devices in your revision area – and where you would remove all distractions in your bedroom.

Highlight three changes you can make at home so that your revision zone stays separate from your sleep zone.

Explain to a partner how each change helps you concentrate when revising and relax when sleeping.

Sleep IS revision

Avoid the all-nighters – sleep is your best revision tool.

We know the pressure is on during exam season – timetables are packed, notes are everywhere, and your brain is juggling more facts than ever. With so much pressure, it can be tempting to burn the candle at both ends and swap sleep for revision. The problem is: skipping sleep to study might actually hurt your performance instead of helping it.

Here are some tips to protect your sleep (and your sanity) during exam season:

Sleep and stress: a two-way street

Stress and sleep are closely connected. When you're stressed, your body produces more cortisol (the stress hormone), which can make it harder to fall asleep or stay asleep. On the flip side, not getting enough sleep increases stress levels. It's like a bad feedback loop – and it can spiral quickly if you're not careful.

Good sleep helps regulate your mood, reduces anxiety, and improves focus. It's one of the most powerful tools you have for managing stress. Think of it as emotional first aid for your brain.

Late-night revision: is it worth it?

We understand – cramming feels productive. But pulling all-nighters or sleeping just a few hours can seriously mess with how your brain works.

Here's what happens when you cut back on sleep to study:

- **Memory gets worse**: Sleep is when your brain sorts and stores what you've learned. Without it, you're more likely to forget things during the exam.

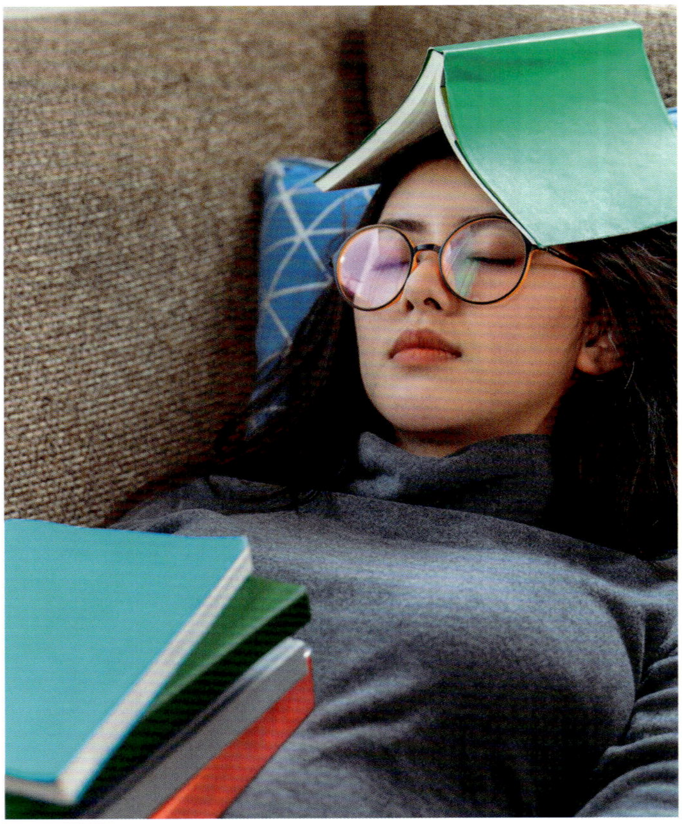

- **Focus drops**: Tired brains are easily distracted and struggle to concentrate.
- **Mood takes a hit**: Sleep-deprived teens are more irritable and anxious – definitely not ideal before a big test.
- **Reaction times slow down**: You might miss key details or make careless mistakes.

Staying up late to revise can backfire. You're better off getting a solid night's sleep.

How to get the sleep you need (even during exams)

You don't need perfect sleep – just better sleep. Here's how to make it happen:

Stick to a schedule

Try to go to bed and wake up at the same time every day– even on weekends. This helps your body clock stay in sync, making it easier to fall asleep and wake up.

Wind down properly

Give yourself 30–60 minutes before bed to chill out. Turn off revision mode and do something relaxing – read, listen to music, stretch, or take a warm shower.

Limit screen time at night

Phones and laptops give off blue light, which tricks your brain into thinking it's still daytime. Try to switch off screens an hour before bed if you can.

Don't revise in bed

Keep your bed for sleeping. If you study in bed, your brain will start to associate it with work – not rest.

Get outside during the day

Natural light helps reset your body clock and improves sleep at night. Even a 20-minute walk outside can make a difference.

Remember: sleep *is* revision

Sleep is when your brain locks in everything you've learned during the day. It's not a waste of time – it's part of your exam prep.

So the next time you feel tempted to keep going past midnight, ask yourself: would I rather study tired and forget, or sleep well and remember?

You've got this!

2025

The above information is reprinted with kind permission from The Sleep Charity.
© 2025 The Sleep Charity

www.teensleephub.org.uk

Sleep training is no longer just for babies. Some schools are teaching teens how to sleep

Sleep training is no longer just for newborns.

By Jocelyn Gecker

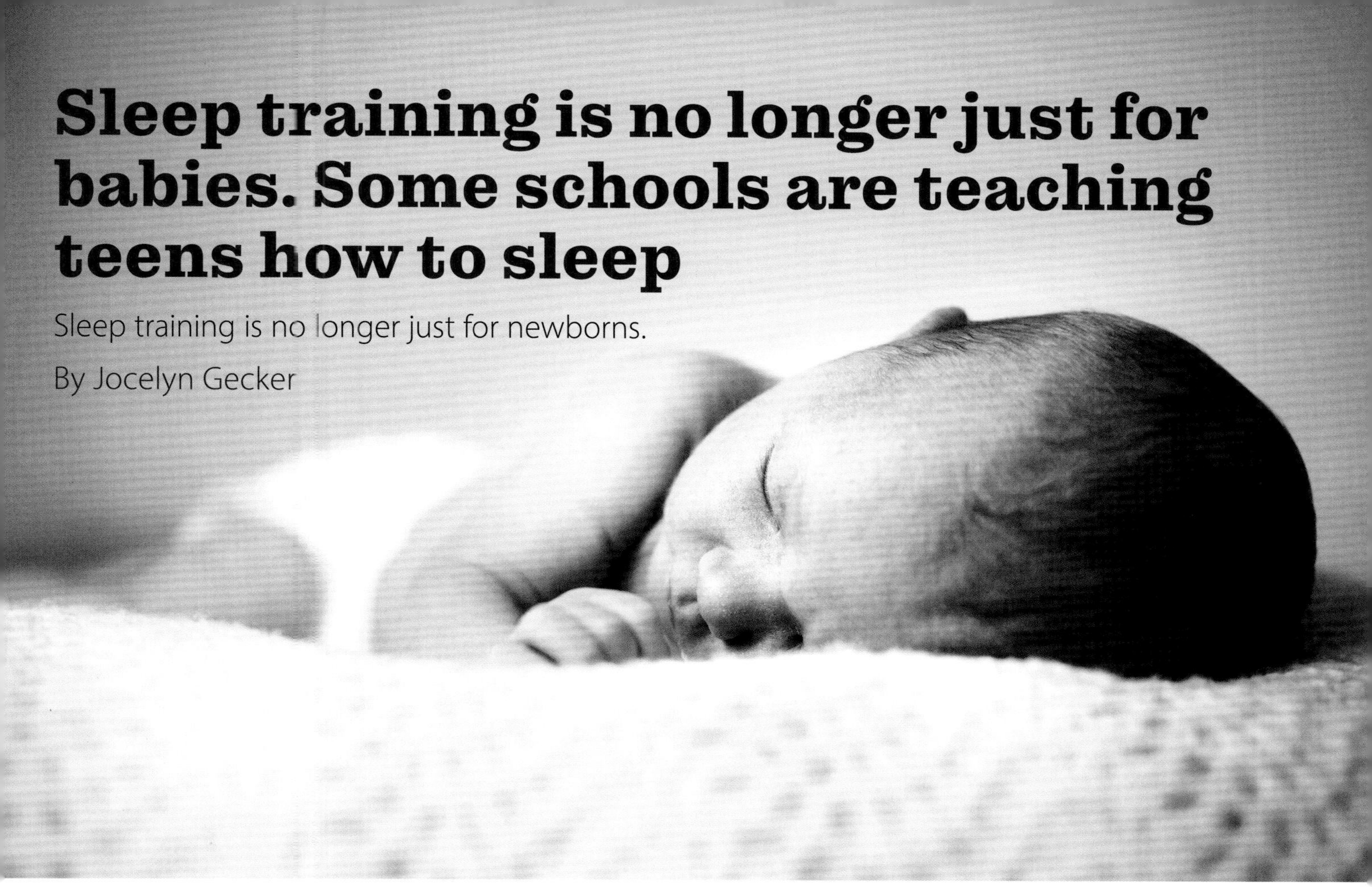

The topic of a new course at Mansfield Senior High School is one that teenagers across the country are having trouble with: How to Get to Sleep.

One ninth grader in the class says his method is to scroll through TikTok until he nods off. Another teen says she often falls asleep while on a late-night group chat with friends. Not everyone takes part in class discussions on a recent Friday; some students are slumped over their desks napping.

Sleep training is no longer just for newborns. Some schools are taking it upon themselves to teach teenagers how to get a good night's sleep.

'It might sound odd to say that kids in high school have to learn the skills to sleep,' says Mansfield health teacher Tony Davis, who has incorporated a newly released sleep curriculum into a state-required high school health class. 'But you'd be shocked how many just don't know how to sleep.'

Adolescents burning the midnight oil is nothing new; teens are biologically programmed to stay up later as their circadian rhythms shift with puberty. But studies show teenagers are more sleep deprived than ever, and experts believe it could be playing a role in the youth mental health crisis and other problems plaguing schools, including behavioural and attendance issues.

'Walk into any high school in America and you will see kids asleep. Whether it's on a desk, outside on the ground or on a bench, or on a couch the school has allotted for naps – because they are exhausted,' says Denise Pope, a senior lecturer at Stanford Graduate School of Education. Pope has surveyed high school students for more than a decade and leads parent sessions for schools around California on the importance of teen sleep. 'Sleep is directly connected with mental health. There is not going to be anyone who argues with that.'

How much sleep do teens need?

Adolescents need between eight and ten hours of sleep each night for their developing brains and bodies. But nearly 80% of teens get less than that, according to the U.S. Centers for Disease Control and Prevention, which has tracked a steady decline in teen sleep since 2007. Today, most teens average six hours of sleep.

Research increasingly shows how tightly sleep is linked to mood, mental health and self-harm. Depression, anxiety and suicidal thoughts and behaviour go up as sleep goes down. Multiple studies also show links between insufficient sleep and sports injuries and athletic performance, teen driving accidents, and risky sexual behaviour and substance use, due in part to impaired judgment when the brain is sleepy.

For years, sleep experts have sounded an alarm about an adolescent sleep crisis, joined by the American Medical Association, the American Academy of Pediatrics, the CDC and others. As a result, some school districts have shifted to later start times. Two states – California and Florida – have passed laws that require high schools to start no earlier than 8:30 a.m. But simply telling a teenager to get to bed earlier

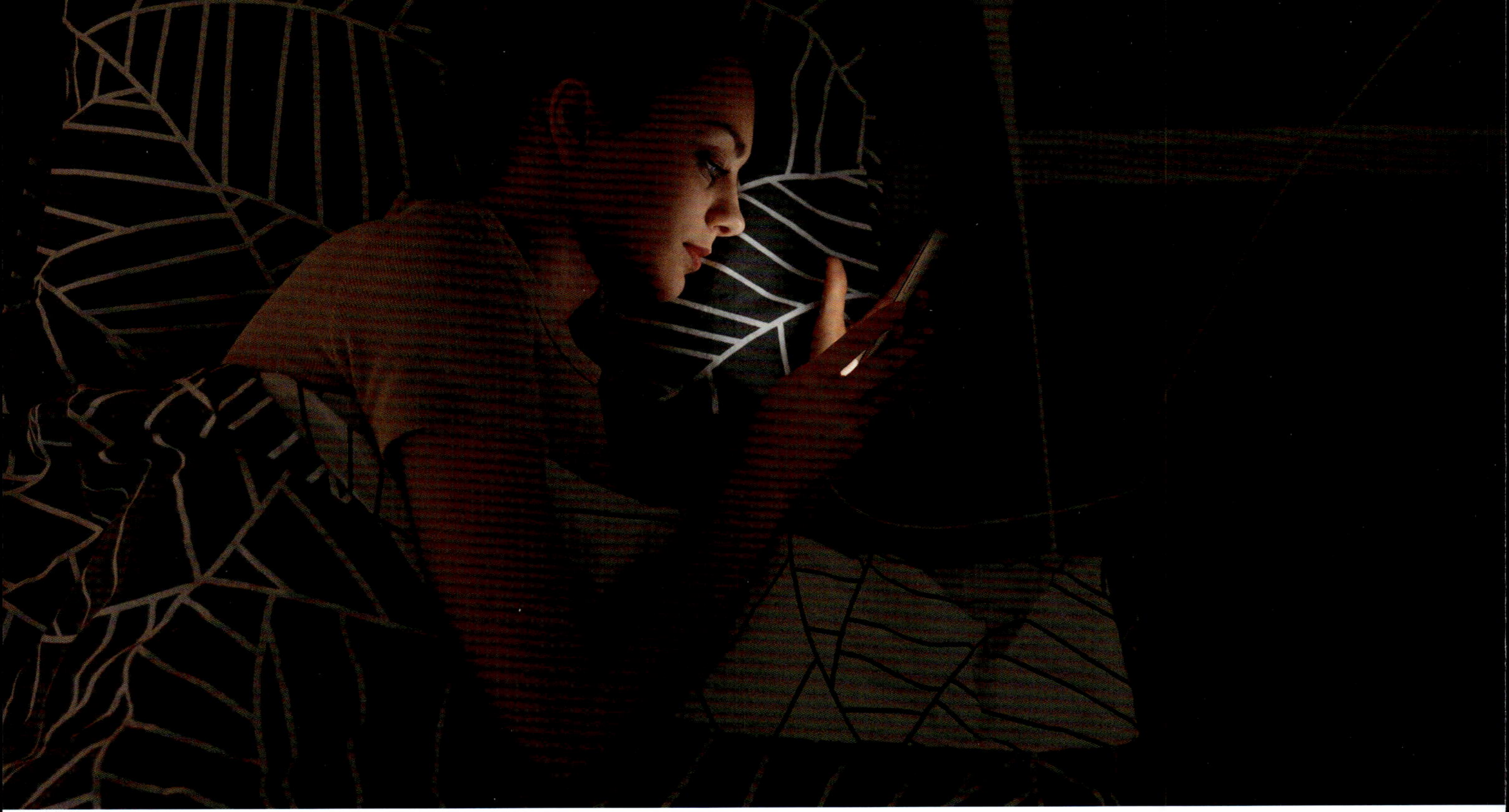

doesn't always work, as any parent can attest: They need to be convinced.

That's why Mansfield City Schools, a district of 3,000 students in north-central Ohio, is staging what it calls 'a sleep intervention.'

'Sleep to Be a Better You'

The district's high school is piloting the new curriculum, 'Sleep to Be a Better You,' hoping to improve academic success and reduce chronic absences, when a student misses more than 10% of the school year. The rate of students missing that much class has decreased from 44% in 2021 but is still high at 32%, says Kari Cawrse, the district's attendance coordinator. Surveys of parents and students highlighted widespread problems with sleep, and an intractable cycle of kids going to bed late, oversleeping, missing the school bus and staying home.

The students in Davis' classroom shared insights into why it's hard to get a good night's sleep. An in-class survey of the 90 students across Davis' five classes found over 60% use their phone as an alarm clock. Over 50% go to sleep while looking at their phones. Experts have urged parents for years to get phones out of the bedroom at night, but national surveys show most teens keep their mobile phones within reach – and many fall asleep holding their devices.

During the six-part course, students are asked to keep daily sleep logs for six weeks and rate their mood and energy levels.

Freshman Nathan Baker assumed he knew how to sleep, but realises he had it all wrong. Bedtime meant settling into bed with his phone, watching videos on YouTube or Snapchat Spotlight and often staying up past midnight. On a good night, he got five hours of sleep. He'd feel so drained by midday that he'd get home and sleep for hours, not realising it was disrupting his nighttime sleep.

'Bad habits definitely start around middle school, with all the stress and drama,' Baker says. He has taken the tips he learned in sleep class and been amazed at the results. He now has a sleep routine that starts around 7 or 8 pm. He puts away his phone for the night and avoids evening snacks, which can disrupt the body's circadian rhythm. He tries for a regular bedtime of 10 pm, making sure to close his curtains and turn off the TV. He likes listening to music to fall asleep but has switched from his previous playlist of rousing hip hop to calmer R&B or jazz, on a stereo instead of his phone.

'I feel a lot better. I'm coming to school with a smile on my face,' says Baker, who is now averaging seven hours' sleep each night. 'Life is so much more simple.'

There are scientific reasons for that. Studies with MRI scans show the brain is under stress when sleep-deprived and functions differently. There is less activity in the pre-frontal cortex, which regulates emotions, decision-making, focus and impulse control and more activity in the emotional centre of the brain, the amygdala, which processes fear, anger and anxiety.

Parents and teens themselves often aren't aware of the signs of sleep deprivation, and attribute it to typical teen behaviour: Being irritable, grumpy, emotionally fragile, unmotivated, impulsive or generally negative.

Think of toddlers who throw temper tantrums when they miss their naps.

'Teenagers have meltdowns, too, because they're tired. But they do it in more age-appropriate ways,' says Kyla Wahlstrom, an adolescent sleep expert at the University of Minnesota, who has studied the benefits of delayed school start times on teen sleep for decades. Wahlstrom developed the free sleep curriculum being used by Mansfield and several Minnesota schools.

Social media isn't only to blame

Social media has been blamed for fuelling the teen mental health crisis, but many experts say the national conversation has ignored the critical role of sleep.

'The evidence linking sleep and mental health is a lot tighter, more causal, than the evidence for social media and mental health,' says Andrew Fuligni, a professor of psychiatry at the University of California, Los Angeles, and co-director at UCLA's Center for the Developing Adolescent.

Nearly 70% of Davis' Mansfield students said they regularly feel sleepy or exhausted during the school day. But technology is hardly the only reason. Today's students are over scheduled, overworked and stressed out, especially as they get closer to senior year and college applications.

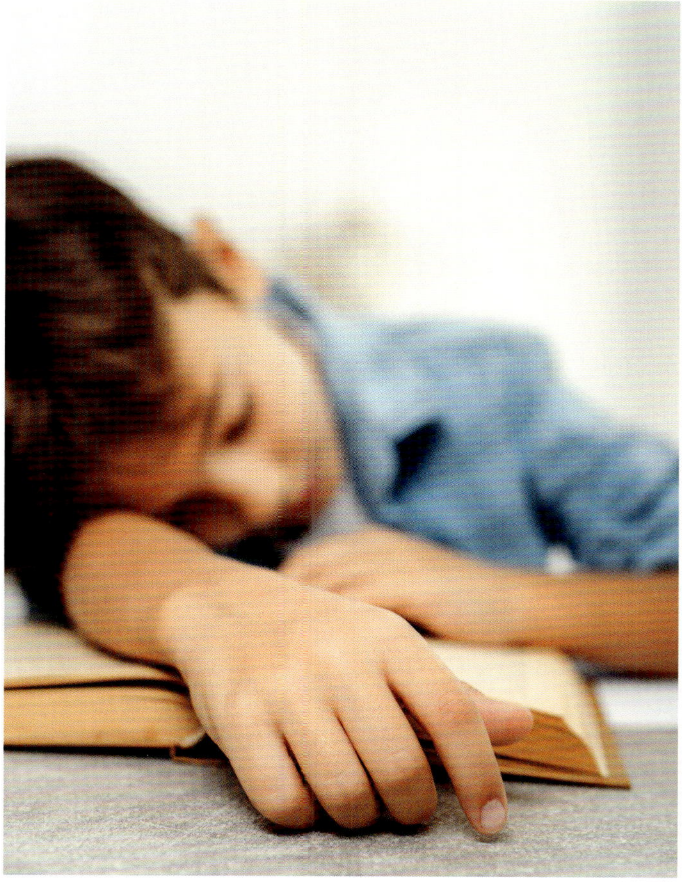

Chase Cole, a senior at Mansfield who is taking three advanced placement and honours classes, is striving for an athletic scholarship to play soccer in college. He plays on three different soccer leagues and typically has practice until 7 pm, when he gets home and needs a nap. Cole wakes up for dinner, then dives into homework for at least three hours. He allows for five-minute phone breaks between assignments and winds down before bed with video games or TV until about 1 am.

'I definitely need to get more sleep at night,' says Cole, 17. 'But it's hard with all my honours classes and college stuff going on. It's exhausting.'

There aren't enough hours in the day to sleep, says sophomore Amelia Raphael, 15. A self-described overachiever, Raphael is taking physics, honours chemistry, algebra and trigonometry and is enrolled in online college classes. Her goal is to finish her associate degree by the time she graduates high school.

'I don't want to have to pay for college. It's a lot of money,' says Raphael, who plays three sports and is in student council and other clubs.

She knows she's over scheduled. 'But if you don't do that, you're kind of setting yourself up for failure. There is a lot of pressure on doing everything,' said Raphael, who gets to bed between midnight and 2 am 'I am giving up sleep for that.'

16 April 2025

The above information is reprinted with kind permission from *The Independent*.
© independent.co.uk 2025

www.independent.co.uk

Personal sleep improvement contract

Reflect on what you've learned about sleep so far.

Write a contract outlining three specific sleep goals for the next month (for example – 'I will switch off all screens by 9 pm').

Include how you will measure success (for example – 'I will record my screen-off time in my sleep log').

Sign and date your contract, then display it on your bedroom wall as a reminder.

Design a classroom nap zone

Imagine your school will set up a supervised nap area with mats or couches.

In pairs, sketch a layout showing where students would rest, store phones and relax.

List three 'nap zone rules' that will prevent distractions and ensure restorative naps (for example – no loud talking, lights dimmed).

Share your design and rules with the class.

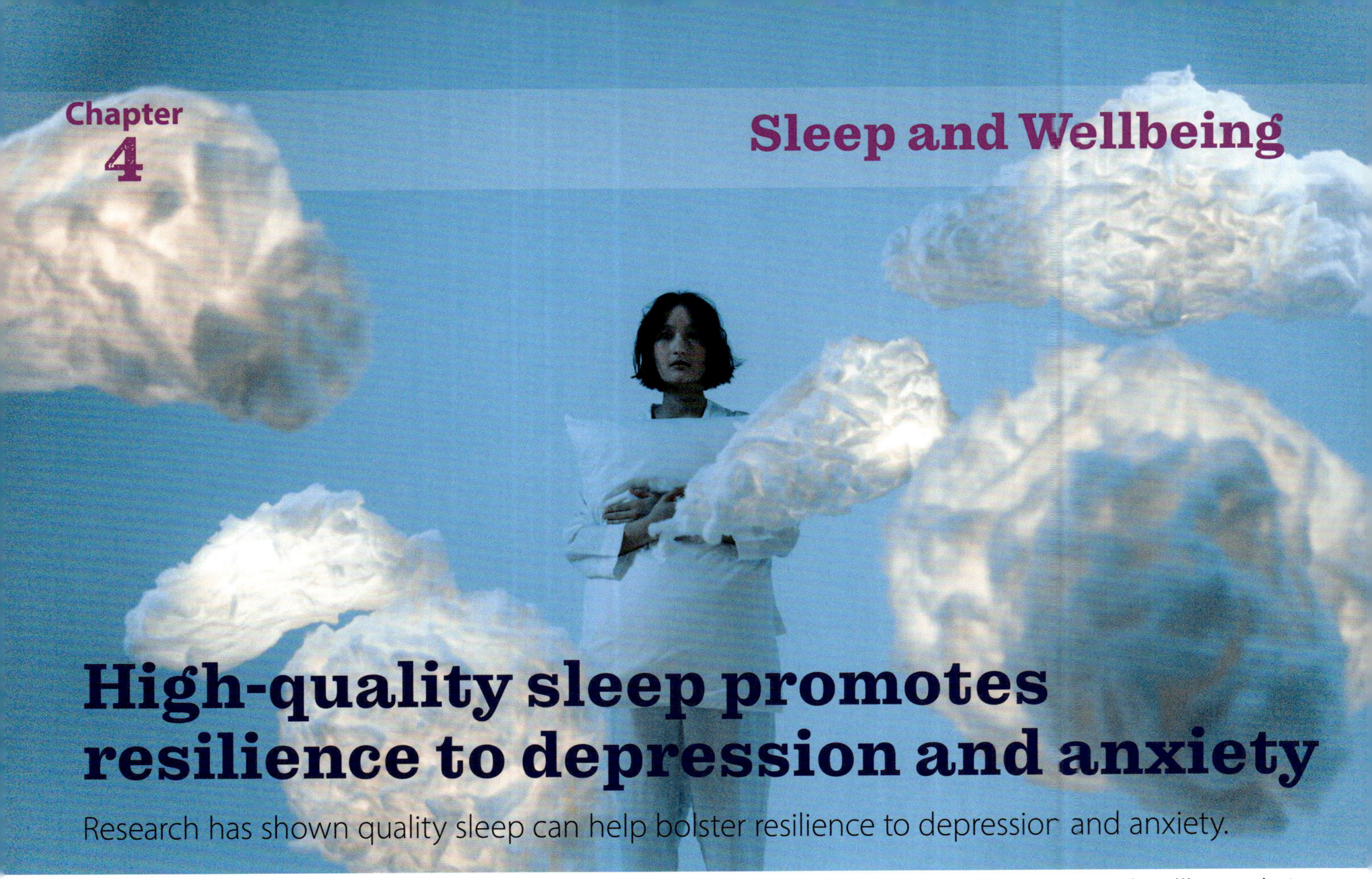

High-quality sleep promotes resilience to depression and anxiety

Research has shown quality sleep can help bolster resilience to depression and anxiety.

The study, led by researchers at the University of York, highlights that chronic stress is a major risk factor for a number of mental health disorders, including depression and pathological anxiety, but high-quality sleep and coping strategies – such as the ability to reframe a situation to see the positive side – can help to prevent poor mental health when faced with negative or stressful experiences.

The research studied data from over 600 participants during the COVID-19 pandemic in 2020 – an extended stressful period of time. They aimed to test the theory that coping strategies supported positive mental health outcomes, which could be strengthened by high-quality sleep.

Unique context

Emma Sullivan, PhD student from the Department of Psychology at the University of York, said: 'As the COVID-19 pandemic has been a prolonged period of stress for people across the entire world, it offered us with a unique context with which to address our research questions.

'This is the first study to investigate the ways in which positive coping strategies and sleep quality influence depression and anxiety when experiencing a real-world chronic stressor. We found that better sleep quality was associated with fewer symptoms of both depression and anxiety during the initial months of the COVID-19 pandemic.

'These findings highlight the importance of targeting both positive coping strategies and sleep quality when enduring periods of chronic stress.'

Mental wellbeing

The team analysed data from the Boston College *Daily Sleep and Well-being* Survey where participants regularly self-reported their sleep quality and mental wellbeing during the pandemic.

They also completed a baseline demographic survey to obtain information such as their age, gender and ethnicity. As well as collecting information on participants' sleep and mental wellbeing, the surveys also collected a wealth of additional information such as participants' alcohol consumption, their quarantine status and physical activity levels.

Coping strategies

Dr Scott Cairney, PhD supervisor on the project from the Department of Psychology and York Biomedical Research Institute at the University of York, said: 'We have known for a long time that high-quality sleep is associated with better health and wellbeing outcomes, but we wanted to know whether this would change if sleep and coping strategies were put under intense and prolonged periods of stress, as it was for so many during the pandemic.'

'We found that sleep plays a hugely important role in the management of chronic stress and can sustain wellbeing over a long period of time, reducing symptoms of depression and anxiety.'

13 July 2023

Published paper on sleep and mental health outcomes during COVID-19 accepted in the journal *Cortex*.

The above information is reprinted with kind permission from the University of York.

© 2025 University of York

www.york.ac.uk

Sleep and mental health

There's a close relationship between sleep and mental health. Living with a mental health problem can affect how well you sleep. And poor sleep can have a negative impact on your mental health.

'During the day, my brain is fuzzy, my memory is noticeably affected. I barely have energy to function.'

Types of sleep problem

Everyone needs sleep, but many of us have problems with it. For example, you might:

- Find it hard to fall asleep, stay asleep or wake up earlier than you'd like to – if this happens regularly, it's known as insomnia
- Have experiences that disturb your sleep, such as panic attacks, flashbacks, nightmares, psychosis, and mania or hypomania
- Find it hard to wake up or get out of bed
- Often feel tired or sleepy – this could be because you're not sleeping enough, not getting good quality sleep or because of health problems
- Sleep a lot, which could include sleeping at times when you want, or need, to be awake

Or you may have other difficulties with sleep that aren't mentioned here.

'When I get depressed, I sleep so much. At its worst it was 18 hours a day, because it was the only way that I could stop thinking and stop my mind from saying awful things to me.'

How sleep problems can affect mental health

If you have problems sleeping, this could make your mental health worse. Or it might cause other problems that impact your mental health.

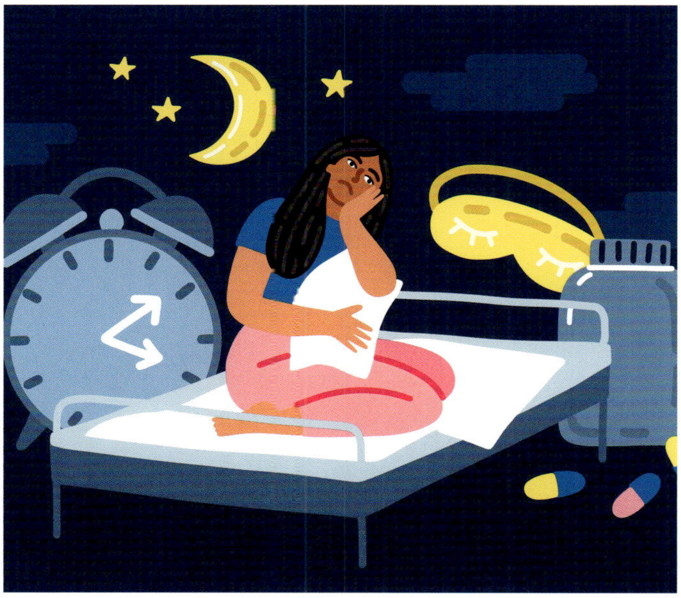

For example, you might:

- Be more likely to feel anxious or depressed
- Be more likely to experience hallucinations
- Be more impacted by symptoms of existing mental health problems, such as mania, psychosis or paranoia
- Feel lonely or isolated – for example, if you don't have the energy to see people, or they don't seem to understand what you're going through
- Struggle to concentrate, or make plans and decisions
- Feel irritable or not have energy to do things
- Have problems with day to day life – for example, at work or with family and friends
- Be more affected by physical health problems

'My sleep problems are more a case of bedtime procrastination than insomnia as such and, as a consequence, being too tired the next morning. I still haven't found out what works for me as I can get to sleep once I do get to bed.'

Causes of sleep problems

The things that affect our sleep differ for everyone. They can include:

- Stresses or worries – for example, issues with money, housing or work
- Problems with where you sleep – for example, if you sleep somewhere uncomfortable or unsafe, or where you're easily disturbed
- Health conditions relating to sleep, also known as sleep disorders
- Being a parent or carer
- Taking medication, including starting or coming off medication
- Using recreational drugs and alcohol
- Working at night or being a shift worker
- Current or past trauma
- Neurodiversity, for example ADHD or autism
- Mental health problems
- Physical health problems

December 2024

The above information is reprinted with kind permission from Mind.

© 2025 Mind

www.mind.org.uk

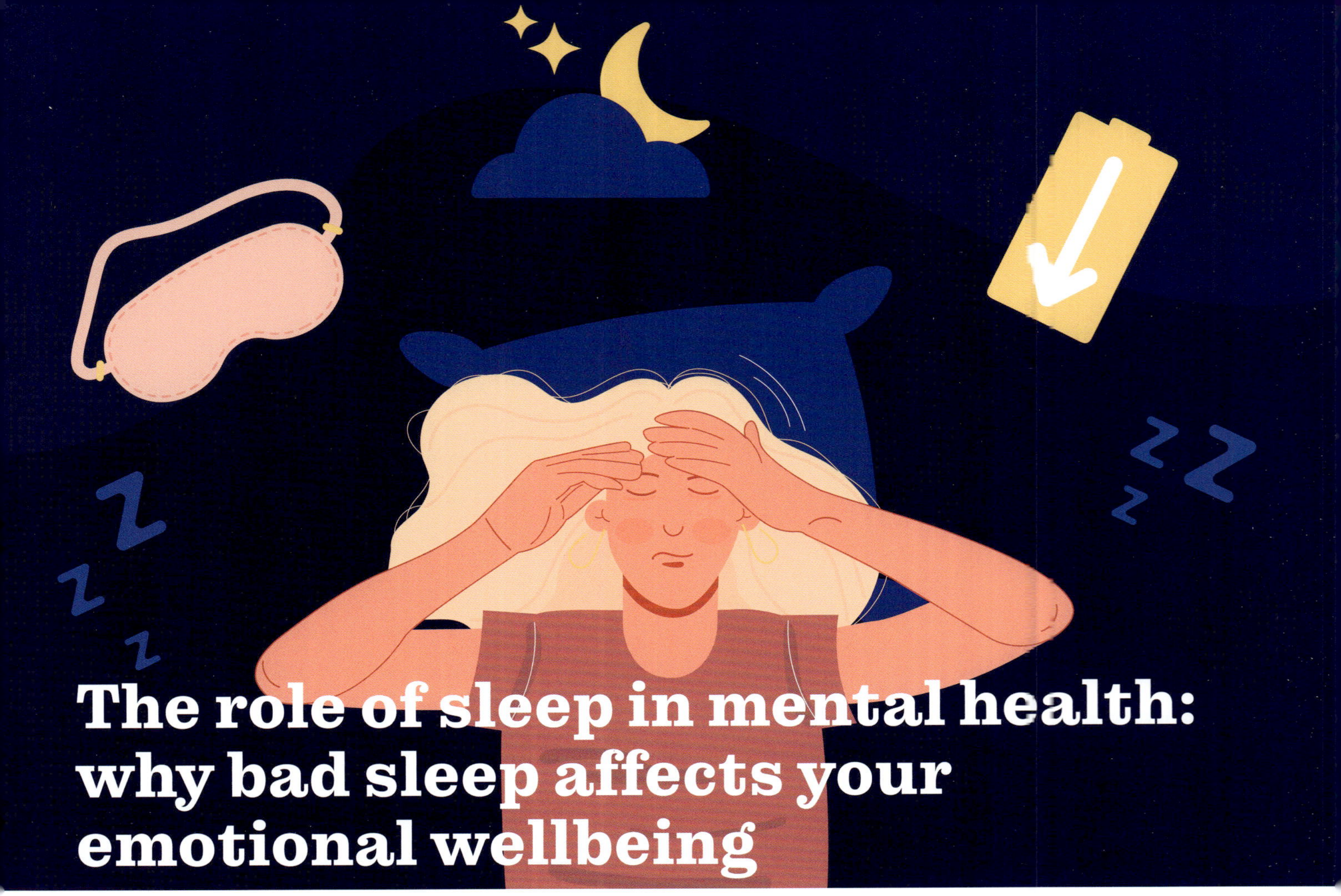

The role of sleep in mental health: why bad sleep affects your emotional wellbeing

We've all had those nights, tossing, turning, staring at the ceiling while the hours creep by. A bad night's sleep leaves us feeling sluggish, irritable, and emotionally drained. But what if poor sleep isn't just an occasional inconvenience? What if it's quietly chipping away at your mental health?

As a humanistic counsellor, I see first-hand how lack of sleep impacts emotional wellbeing. Many clients seek therapy for anxiety, low mood, or feeling overwhelmed only to realise that their sleep patterns are at the heart of the issue. So, why is sleep so crucial, and what can we do about it?

Why sleep matters for mental health

Sleep is essential for processing emotions, consolidating memories, and maintaining psychological resilience. When we sleep well, we wake up refreshed, better able to cope with stress, and more in tune with our emotions. Conversely, a lack of sleep disrupts these vital processes, leaving us more vulnerable to emotional distress.

During deep sleep, the brain processes the events of the day, helping us make sense of our emotions and experiences. This is why we often wake up with a clearer perspective after a good night's rest. Without adequate sleep, our ability to regulate emotions diminishes, increasing the likelihood of feeling overwhelmed, anxious, or irritable. Sleep deprivation also impairs cognitive function, reducing our ability to focus and solve problems effectively.

The link between poor sleep and mental health

Chronic sleep deprivation or insomnia isn't just about feeling tired. It can significantly impact our mental and emotional wellbeing:

Increased anxiety – Poor sleep can make anxiety worse by heightening our brain's reactivity to stress. When we're tired, small worries can spiral into overwhelming concerns. Sleep deprivation increases activity in the amygdala, the part of the brain responsible for fear and anxiety, making it harder to keep emotions in check.

Lowered mood – Sleep and depression are closely linked. A lack of restorative sleep can contribute to persistent low mood and even exacerbate symptoms of clinical depression. Sleep disruptions affect neurotransmitter levels, such as serotonin and dopamine, which play a crucial role in maintaining mood stability.

Emotional reactivity – Ever noticed how everything feels harder after a bad night's sleep? Sleep deprivation affects our ability to regulate emotions, making us more irritable and reactive. Research shows that sleep-deprived individuals have stronger emotional responses to negative experiences, increasing feelings of frustration and sadness.

Difficulty thinking clearly – Poor sleep impacts concentration, problem-solving, and memory. This can make work, relationships, and decision-making feel much more challenging. Lack of sleep affects the prefrontal cortex, the brain region responsible for logical thinking, leading to impaired judgment and increased impulsivity.

Humanistic counselling and the holistic approach to sleep issues

From a humanistic perspective, sleep issues aren't just physical, they're emotional and psychological too. We don't just treat the symptoms; we explore what's really going on underneath. Our thoughts, emotions, and behaviours are interconnected, and identifying the root causes of sleep disturbances is key to improving overall wellbeing.

For example, one client struggled with insomnia and found himself awake every night at 3 am. When we explored his thoughts and feelings, it turned out that unresolved work stress was keeping his mind racing. Through counselling, he identified the pressures he was placing on himself and worked towards more self-compassionate thinking, which ultimately improved his sleep.

Many individuals experiencing sleep problems may also have underlying emotional wounds or unresolved trauma. Addressing these concerns in therapy can help them create a more peaceful mental state, making it easier to relax and achieve restful sleep.

Practical tips for better sleep and mental wellbeing

If you're struggling with sleep and it's affecting your mental health, here are some practical, humanistic approaches you can try:

Create a sleep-friendly environment

- Keep your bedroom dark, cool, and quiet. Use blackout curtains, earplugs, or a white noise machine if necessary.
- Avoid screens at least an hour before bed (blue light messes with melatonin production, the hormone that regulates sleep).
- Invest in a comfortable mattress and pillows that support restful sleep.

Establish a pre-sleep routine

- Try reading, journaling, or gentle stretching before bed. Engaging in calming activities signals to the brain that it's time to wind down.
- Avoid overstimulating activities like scrolling social media or watching intense TV shows. High-stimulation content can keep your mind engaged and delay sleep onset.
- Develop a consistent bedtime schedule by going to bed and waking up at the same time every day, even on weekends.

Mind your thoughts

- If your mind races at night, try a 'brain dump'. Write down worries before bed to get them out of your head. This technique can prevent ruminative thinking that disrupts sleep.
- Practice mindfulness or deep breathing to ease an anxious mind. Guided meditation or progressive muscle relaxation can help you unwind.
- Challenge negative thought patterns that may be contributing to stress and sleep difficulties. Cognitive restructuring techniques can help reframe anxious thoughts in a more balanced way.

Listen to your body

- If you're not sleepy, don't force sleep. Get up, do something relaxing, and return to bed when you feel tired.
- Avoid caffeine, nicotine, or heavy meals too close to bedtime, as they can interfere with your body's natural sleep cycle.
- Engage in regular physical activity during the day, but avoid vigorous exercise close to bedtime as it can be too stimulating.

Address underlying emotional issues

- Counselling can help uncover hidden anxieties or stresses contributing to poor sleep. Exploring emotional concerns in therapy can provide clarity and relief.
- Talking through concerns with a therapist can ease the mental load that keeps you awake at night. Expressing emotions in a safe space can reduce psychological tension and improve sleep quality.
- Consider exploring self-compassion practices to counteract self-criticism and internalised stress that may be affecting your ability to rest.

Final thoughts

Bad sleep and mental health go hand in hand. If you're struggling with emotional wellbeing, examining your sleep habits could be a vital step towards feeling better. Humanistic counselling offers a compassionate, holistic way to explore what's really going on beneath the surface because sometimes, the key to a better night's sleep isn't just about bedtime routines, but about how we process our emotions throughout the day.

If sleep is affecting your mental health, you don't have to suffer in silence. Seeking support can help you regain balance, both in your nights and in your waking life.

13 February 2025

The above information is reprinted with kind permission from George Fortune Counselling.
© 2025 George Fortune Counselling

www.georgefortunecounselling.co.uk

The negative effects of sleep deprivation on body and mind

By Rachel Ayre

Sleep is a fundamental human need, essential for maintaining optimal physical and mental health. Despite its importance, many people consistently fail to get the recommended amount of sleep. The NHS recommends that adults aim for 7–9 hours of sleep per night, with some individuals benefiting from 8+ hours to function optimally. However, modern lifestyles often interfere with achieving this goal, leading to widespread sleep deprivation. Here, we explore the detrimental effects of sleep deprivation on both body and mind, and provide advice for those struggling with insomnia.

Physical repercussions of sleep deprivation

Lack of sleep can have immediate and long-term effects on the body. Here are some of the key physical repercussions:

- Impaired immune function: Sleep is crucial for the proper functioning of the immune system. Chronic sleep deprivation can weaken the immune response, making the body more susceptible to infections and illnesses. Studies have shown that individuals who sleep less than 7 hours per night are nearly three times more likely to develop a cold, compared to those who sleep 8 hours or more.
- Weight gain and obesity: Insufficient sleep disrupts the balance of hormones that regulate hunger and appetite, such as ghrelin and leptin. This imbalance can lead to increased hunger and cravings for high-calorie foods, contributing to weight gain and obesity. Additionally, sleep deprivation affects insulin sensitivity, increasing the risk of type 2 diabetes.
- Cardiovascular health: Sleep is vital for heart health. Chronic sleep deprivation is associated with an increased risk of hypertension, heart disease, and stroke. Research indicates that sleeping less than 6 hours per night is linked to a 48% increased risk of developing or dying from coronary heart disease and a 15% increased risk of stroke.
- Reduced physical performance: Lack of sleep impairs physical performance by reducing muscle strength, endurance, and reaction times. Athletes and physically active individuals who do not get enough sleep are more prone to injuries and have longer recovery times.

Mental repercussions of sleep deprivation

Sleep deprivation also significantly impacts mental health and cognitive function. The following are some key mental repercussions:

- Cognitive impairment: Sleep is essential for cognitive processes such as attention, learning, memory, and problem-solving. Sleep-deprived individuals often experience difficulties with concentration, decision-making, and retaining information. Chronic sleep deprivation has been linked to a decline in

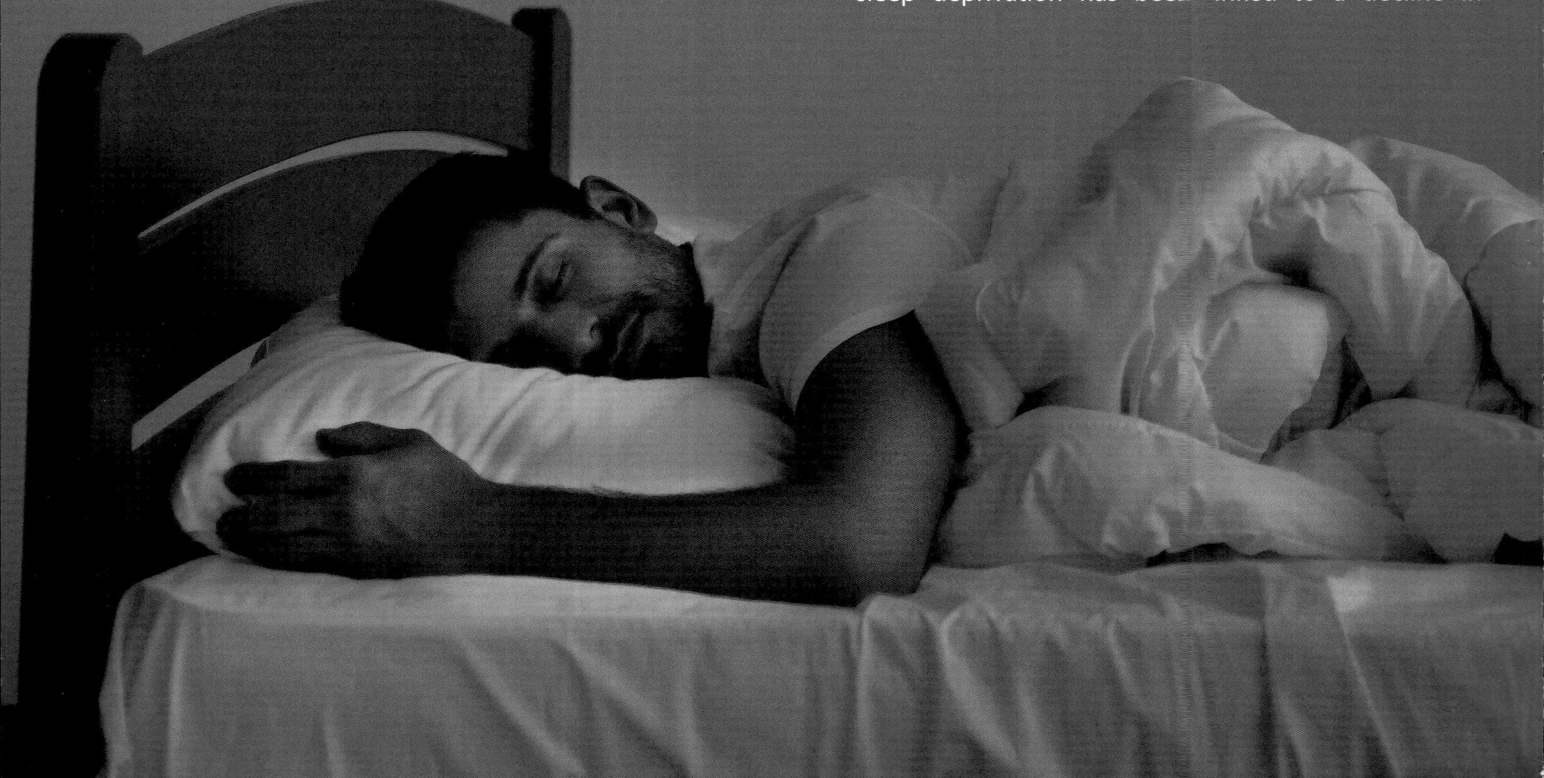

overall cognitive function, and an increased risk of neurodegenerative diseases, such as Alzheimer's.

- Mood disorders: Lack of sleep can negatively affect mood and emotional regulation. Sleep-deprived individuals are more likely to experience irritability, anxiety, and depression. In fact, insomnia is a common symptom and predictor of mood disorders, with chronic sleep problems significantly increasing the risk of developing depression.
- Mental health disorders: Sleep deprivation can exacerbate symptoms of existing mental health conditions such as anxiety disorders, bipolar disorder, and schizophrenia. Moreover, chronic sleep problems can contribute to the development of new mental health issues.
- Decreased quality of life: Persistent sleep deprivation affects overall quality of life, reducing one's ability to engage in daily activities and enjoy life. This can lead to a cycle of poor sleep and reduced life satisfaction, further impacting mental health.

Importance of sleep for health

Sleep plays a critical role in maintaining health and wellbeing. Here are some ways in which sufficient sleep benefits us:

- Restoration and repair: Sleep allows the body to repair muscles, tissues, and cells. It also supports growth and development in children and adolescents.
- Cognitive function: Sleep enhances brain function, including memory consolidation, learning, and problem-solving skills.
- Emotional regulation: Adequate sleep helps regulate emotions and reduces the risk of mood disorders.
- Immune function: Quality sleep strengthens the immune system, helping the body fight off infections and illnesses.

Advice for people struggling with insomnia

For those struggling with insomnia, the following tips may help improve sleep quality:

1. Maintain a consistent sleep schedule: Go to bed and wake up at the same time every day, even on weekends. This helps regulate the body's internal clock.
2. Create a relaxing bedtime routine: Engage in calming activities before bed, such as reading, meditating, or taking a warm bath. Avoid stimulating activities like using electronic devices, watching TV, or working.
3. Optimise your sleep environment: Ensure your bedroom is conducive to sleep. Keep the room dark, quiet, and cool. Invest in a comfortable mattress and pillows.
4. Limit caffeine and alcohol: Avoid consuming caffeine and alcohol close to bedtime, as they can interfere with sleep.
5. Exercise regularly: Regular physical activity can promote better sleep, but avoid vigorous exercise close to bedtime.
6. Seek professional help: If insomnia persists despite trying these strategies, consider consulting a healthcare professional or sleep specialist. Cognitive-behavioural therapy (CBT) for insomnia is an effective treatment for chronic sleep problems.

Conclusion

Sleep deprivation has profound negative effects on both the body and mind, compromising overall health and wellbeing. By prioritising sleep and adopting healthy sleep habits, you can improve your physical and mental health, enhancing your quality of life. Remember, getting enough sleep is not a luxury, but a necessity for a healthy, fulfilling life.

11 July 2024

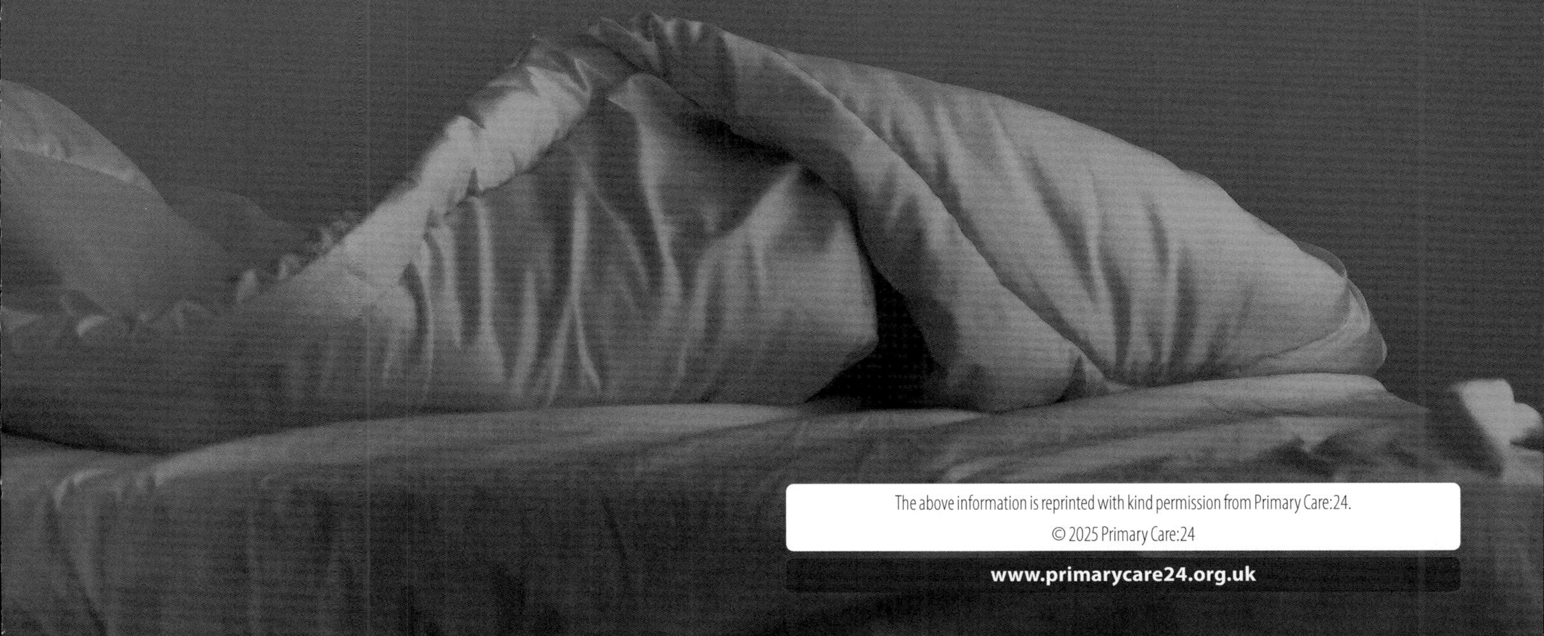

The above information is reprinted with kind permission from Primary Care:24.
© 2025 Primary Care:24
www.primarycare24.org.uk

What having a power nap does for your health

A short snatch of sleep in the day can kick-start the brain and boost alertness. But how much is too much?

By Jenny Tucker

My relationship with sleep is tenuous. It often eludes me, and so I spend my waking hours in a half-trance while blathering on about how shattered I feel. Meanwhile, one of my best friends announces she regularly 'micro' naps. It's a shiny new term, used in favour of the 1990s 'power' nap label, which emerged after a study on sleep-ravaged American pilots revealed that if they napped before long-haul flights they were more alert at the end of the trip.

My friend closes her eyes for fragments of time throughout the day to boost her endurance so she can cope with the minefield of being a working mother of five. She says it gives her the necessary kick that no amount of caffeine can ever achieve.

Research agrees she is on to something. Napping has been shown to improve cognitive and emotional health, with many sleep experts I have interviewed saying around 10 minutes is the optimum amount of shut eye. Even Real Madrid have made their bed to lie in it. As part of the team's training regimen, they've adopted an afternoon siesta routine to help optimise performance and quick recovery. Then there's Google and Nike, who reportedly have sleep 'pods' and 'quiet' rooms for napping and meditation to facilitate their wearier employees. PJs optional.

So perhaps I've been getting it wrong all this time. Rather than craving an endless stretch of night time REM, maybe I should be losing myself in slithers of rejuvenating daytime dozing? Should we all be doing this to improve our health?

What are the health benefits of a power nap?

Dr Guy Meadows, a sleep psychologist, author and founder of The Sleep School, believes there are many health benefits to taking a short snatch of sleep during the day.

'When we nap, the body and brain enter light sleep, helping to restore energy, improve memory, reduce stress and support heart and cognitive health. Napping may offer cardiovascular benefits, especially for people who are sleep-deprived or under stress. Some studies have found that short naps can lower blood pressure and reduce heart rate variability, promoting heart health. Naps boost memory consolidation, emotional regulation, and problem-solving.'

Dr Meadows also believes that naps may indirectly help with 'weight regulation by reducing fatigue-driven snacking.' Good news to all late-night snackers.

One study by researchers at University College London (UCL) focused on participants aged between 40 and 69 and found that those who habitually napped had larger brain volume – an indication that regular short sleep aids better overall brain health by slowing the rate at which the brain shrinks with age, potentially helping to lower risk of dementia and other diseases.

It's also a plus when it comes to creative thinking. The brain needs periods of rest to improve its problem-solving capability and build fresh ideas. Additionally, in those who are sleep deprived, high levels of the stress hormone cortisol can fester, so closing your eyes, even for a limited time, can alleviate a sense of overwhelm.

What's the right amount of napping?

Experts say anything between 10–20 minutes is best; anything longer can have a detrimental effect.

Dr Maja Schaedel, the co-founder of The Good Sleep Clinic, adds: 'We know that just a 15-minute nap can help our bodies go through a process of improvement – our tissues are repaired, muscle grows and our immune system is strengthened. Napping is extremely good when learning new skills and in infants it's vital.'

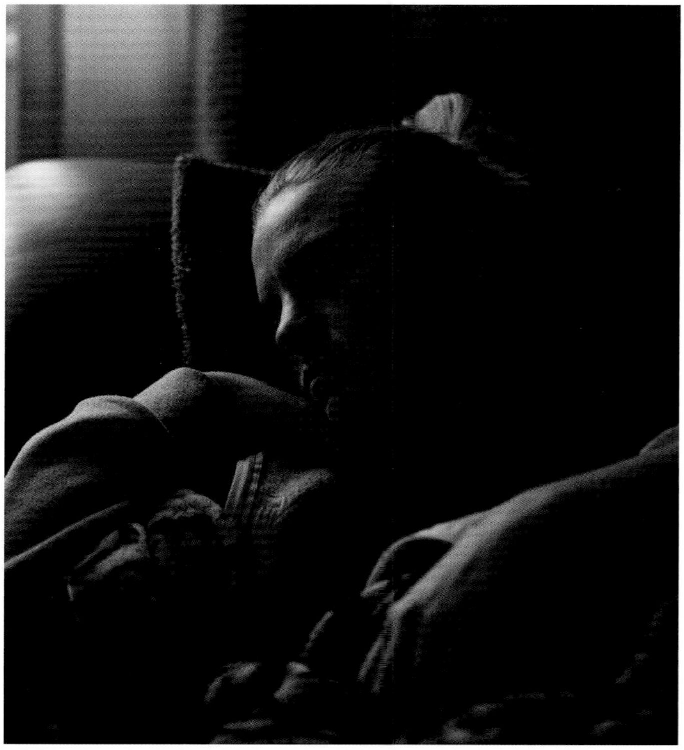

What are the negatives of napping?

There can be negatives to a power nap if they go on too long or are indulged too frequently.

Dr David Lee, a clinical director at Sleep Unlimited and author of *Teaching the World to Sleep*, is somewhat sceptical.

'In a healthy sleeper, who is getting enough good quality sleep at night, napping isn't generally a thing,' he explains. 'If someone came to me and said they were napping a lot, I'd want to look at their overall sleep patterns. The problem is, if you nap during the day, you are going to reduce some of your sleep pressure [the drive to sleep that builds up the longer you're awake, and is mainly regulated by adenosine, a chemical that accumulates in your brain throughout the day] and that may mean more difficulty dropping off at night or sleeping through.'

So, although feeling tired can seem like a drag, it's an essential part of our body clock. Ideally, we want the sleep pressure to accumulate so that when we reach the end of our day, we want nothing more than to be horizontal under the duvet.

Dr Schaedel points out: 'Napping during the day can be disruptive to your night rest, which can result in a vicious cycle. The more night time awakenings we have, the more tired you feel the next day and so the more you will be inclined to nap again.'

Dr Lee makes it simple: 'If you can nap during the day and still manage a good night's sleep, then go ahead. If not, cut out the naps. I work with loads of people who have trouble sleeping, but the worst sleeper in the world will sleep well if you keep them awake for a significant amount of time. They will build up shed loads of sleep pressure and ultimately need to close their eyes.'

Is it for everyone?

Like most habits, it's not a one size fits all. Some people, like my friend, can sleep for England during the day and still kip at night. But others may find that napping messes with their sleep pressure and circadian system (the internal clock that regulates sleep-wake cycles), forcing them to stare wildly at the ceiling into the wee hours.

It is no surprise that anyone who suffers with insomnia should avoid napping.

'There are certain groups who can benefit' says Dr Lee. 'Much older people, those with a brain injury, anyone who has suffered a stroke or dementia patients may find a nap is neuro protective. But I'd still recommend keeping it short, no more than two hours'

Should we all take more naps as we age?

Studies show that around 25% of the over-60s take daytime naps. But while it can help improve alertness, frequent daytime napping can indicate underlying health issues.

Russell Foster, a professor of circadian neuroscience, writes in his book, *Life Time*: 'There is an assumption that older people need less sleep, or are incapable of getting good sleep, but neither of these assumptions may be true. Aged individuals generally take longer to sleep, and experience more broken sleep, and shorter night-time sleep. All this leads to an increased likelihood of daytime naps. But this is not a problem unless it affects your daytime ability to function.'

Perhaps the bottom line is, if you enjoy a nap and find it reviving, good for you. If you need a nap because you're depleted and can't fully function without it, consider what else might be going on and if it's time to get your GP involved.

FAQs

Can I nap for more than 20 minutes if I need it?

If you stick within the 10–20 minute boundary, having a brief doze shouldn't interrupt your night-time routine. Carry on snoozing, and your sleep pressure will be compromised.

How close to bedtime should I nap?

Dr Meadows says: 'A short sleep taken before 3pm won't harm your normal routine and may even help make up for lost rest.' Winston Churchill famously slept for an hour or two at 4.30pm after a late lunch, but he was a confirmed night owl and often didn't go to bed until the early hours.

What if I fall asleep in the evening watching TV?

Not the best idea. Again, if it's a limited nod, you may get away with it. But it's often better to push through the drowsiness and have an early night rather than a late nap.

How can I make sure I don't oversleep on my nap?

Set an alarm (coming round to gentle music is a good idea), nap in a room that is cool in temperature and semi-lit, sit in a chair rather than go to bed, and stick to a napping routine (same time, same place) to train your body to wake up naturally.

At what age should I stop napping?

It's not about age. If it works, even with much older people, continue. Reasons to stop are more around disrupted sleep at night, or if a nap leaves you feeling groggy and at risk when carrying out tasks like driving, managing stairs or using certain household appliances

20 April 2025

The above information is reprinted with kind permission from *The Telegraph*.
© Telegraph Media Group Limited 2025

www.telegraph.co.uk

Useful Websites

Useful websites

www.drsandipbanerjee.co.uk

www.georgefortunecounselling.co.uk

www.independent.co.uk

www.londondaily.news

www.mentalhealth.org.uk

www.mind.org.uk

www.nhs.uk

www.primarycare24.org.uk

www.surrey.ac.uk

www.teenagementalhealth.co.uk

www.teensleephub.org.uk

www.telegraph.co.uk

www.theconversation.com

www.theinsomniaclinic.co.uk

www.york.ac.uk

www.yougov.co.uk

Glossary

Blue light
A type of light from screens that helps with alertness during the day but can make it harder to sleep if used too close to bedtime.

Bruxism
A condition where someone grinds their teeth while asleep. It's often linked to stress or anxiety.

Caffeine
A natural stimulant found in tea, coffee and some soft drinks that can make people feel more awake or alert.

Circadian rhythm
The body's internal clock that controls when we feel sleepy or awake across a 24-hour day.

Cognitive behavioural therapy (CBT)
A talking therapy that helps people understand and change unhelpful thoughts and behaviours.

Deep sleep
A stage of sleep when the body repairs itself and you're hardest to wake.

Digital detox
A break from social media or digital devices to reduce stress or regain focus.

Dreams
Stories, images or feelings that the brain creates during sleep.

FOMO
Fear of missing out – a feeling of anxiety that others are having fun without you, often caused by social media.

Insomnia
A sleep disorder where it's hard to fall asleep, stay asleep or get good-quality rest.

Jet lag
Tiredness and confusion caused by travelling across time zones and disrupting your body clock.

Light sleep
The first stage of sleep where you drift in and out and can be woken easily.

Medication
Drugs used to treat health conditions. For mental illness, it may be used alongside talking therapies.

Melatonin
A hormone the body makes at night to help you feel sleepy and ready for bed.

Narcolepsy
A rare condition where a person suddenly falls asleep at inappropriate times.

Night terror
A sleep disorder where someone wakes suddenly in fear, often with no memory of it happening.

Nightmare
A scary or upsetting dream that can wake you up and leave you feeling anxious.

Oversleeping
Sleeping for longer than needed, which can sometimes make you feel groggy or low.

Physical activity
Any movement like walking, sport or gardening that helps improve physical and mental health.

Power nap
A short nap (10–20 minutes) that can help boost energy and focus during the day.

Rapid eye movement (REM)
A deep sleep stage where the eyes move quickly and dreaming is most likely to occur.

Restless legs syndrome
A condition where you feel a strong urge to move your legs at night, which can disturb sleep.

Screen time
The amount of time spent using devices like phones, tablets or computers.

Sleep apnoea
A sleep disorder where breathing stops and starts during the night, often causing tiredness.

Sleep cycle
The pattern of sleep stages that repeat during the night, including light sleep, deep sleep and REM sleep.

Sleep deprivation
Not getting enough sleep, which can affect mood, memory and concentration.

Sleep environment
Your sleeping space – things like noise, light, and temperature that can affect how well you sleep.

Sleep hygiene
Healthy habits or routines before bed that help improve sleep quality.

Sleep tracker
A device or app that monitors your sleep patterns and gives feedback on sleep quality.

Sleepwalking
A sleep disorder where a person walks or does other activities while still asleep.

Index